BRAIN, MIND, AND MEDICINE

BRAIN, MIND, AND MEDICINE

Charles Richet and the Origins of Physiological Psychology

Stewart Wolf

Transaction Publishers
New Brunswick (U.S.A.) and London (U.K.)

Library of Congress Catalog Number: 92-1302
ISBN: 1-56000-063-5
Printed in the United States of America

Library of Congress Cataloging-in-Publication Data

Wolf, Stewart, 1914-
    Brain, mind, and medicine: Charles Richet and the origins of physiological psychology / Stewart Wolf.
        p.   cm.
Includes bibliographical references and index.
    ISBN 1-56000-063-5
    1. Richet, Charles Robert, 1850-1935. 2. Physiologists—France—Biography. I. Title
QP26.R5W65   1992
591.1'092—dc20
[B]
                                                        92-1302
                                                          CIP

Contents

Family Tree

Four Generations of Richet Professors at the Faculté de Médecine of Paris

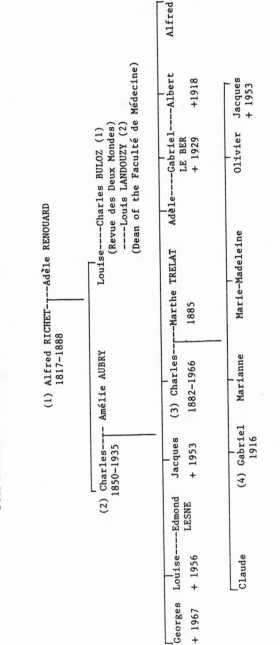

Tables

Preface

Charles Richet was by no means typical of the more than 150 medical scientists who have been awarded the Nobel Prize in physiology or medicine. Most of them had focused their work sharply on a specific unsolved scientific problem and a surprising number of them had studied under and worked closely with mentors who themselves had won the Nobel Prize. They were then likely to continue the line of inquiry of their chiefs. Richet, a free spirit, was not drawn to pursue further the projects of the three world famous teachers in whose laboratories he worked. In fact, he never published in collaboration with any of them. Richet, who studied whatever intrigued him, worked on a variety of seemingly disparate projects. His attention moved like a scanner, sensitive to clues from a wide range of topics. One of his discoveries (not the best one in his mind) happened to qualify for the Nobel Prize but his interest lay not so much in anaphylaxis for which he won the prize, but in a variety of adaptive responses, mainly involving the nervous system, that seemed to afford protection against an adverse environment. These seemingly disparate inquiries led him to a concept about what he called, "the defense of the organism."

Richet, also unlike all but a handful of his fellow Nobel laureates, was a product of a wealthy and prominent family. He savored his freedom and indulged his whims and passions for writing, fishing, and traveling and spent long periods away from his work. Even when at home he usually spent less than half a day in the laboratory while deeply involving himself in a variety of pursuits that to him, like the physiological phenomena he studied, had significance toward protecting not only the human organism but also the human race, the French in particular and mankind in general. His other causes included social justice, eugenics and Esperanto. Notwithstanding his role as paladin, Richet published more than 700 papers in scientific journals. Meanwhile, away from his work at the University and his causes, he wrote novels, plays, and poetry. Two of his poems were recognized by awards from the Académie Française.

Richet's interest in psychology, especially hypnosis, began when he was a youth and continued throughout his life. As he considered psychology to be part of physiology, the central nervous system played a prominent part in most of his physiological research. He treated hysteria with hypnosis on Charcot's service at the Salpêtrière and considered psychology to be part of physiology. His monograph, *Essai de Psychologie Générale*, published in 1885 and translated into several languages, considered psychology as a neural science. In it he dealt not only with stimuli and responses but with memory, consciousness, and ideation.

I first encountered Charles Richet's name in the medical literature in 1941, six years after his death. While studying a patient with a large gastric fistula, an opening into the stomach through the skin of the abdomen, I was searching in the library for reports of others who had had similar opportunities to make direct observations of the inside of the human stomach (Wolf & Wolff 1943). I discovered that Charles Richet, when a recent graduate of the Faculté de Médecine in Paris, had added to discoveries about the human stomach made forty years earlier by the world famous U.S. Army surgeon, William Beaumont, on the stomach of his patient and subject, Alexis St. Martin (Beaumont 1833). St. Martin had sustained a gunshot wound to the abdomen that left him with a gastric fistula. Richet's subject of study was a young man named Marcellin who had a surgically induced similar gastric fistula.[R 14,15.]

In the early 1960s I came across Richet's work again while investigating the "dive reflex," a phylogenetically ancient physiological adaptation that protects an animal against lack of oxygen during breath-hold diving (Wolf 1965, 1966). By slowing the heart rate and shunting blood away from muscles and internal organs except the brain, the adaptive "dive reflex" conserves oxygen still present in the body. Richet, in experiments on diving ducks, had made the first step forward toward understanding the mechanism of this protective phenomenon.[R385] Later, while exploring various mechanisms of sudden death, I experimented with anaphylaxis, an often suddenly fatal sensitivity reaction to a foreign substance (Wolf 1968), and learned that Charles Richet had been awarded the Nobel Prize in 1913 for the discovery of anaphylaxis.[R 543]

By this time I had become as interested in learning about Richet, the man, as in reviewing his work. I was intrigued by his restless curiosity, his wide range of interests and his extraordinary versatility. During a sabbatical year in Paris in 1963–64, I met Richet's son Charles *fils* and his grandson Gabriel. Both were members of the Faculté de Médecine of the University of Paris. In talking with them and with several senior French scientists I was able to learn more about Charles, père, including the fact that, although his career is the subject of a penetrating review in the *Dictionary of Scientific Biography* (Holmes 1975), he had not as yet been the subject of a full biography. Therefore, determined to attempt the task, I bought all of the monographs and journal papers by and about Richet that were available in the bookstores in Paris. Since then I have been able to enlarge my collection and have also studied in the large medical libraries of the eastern United States, and in the Bibliothèque Nationale and the libraries of the Faculté de Médecine and the Académie des Sciences in Paris.

Charles' grandson, Gabriel Richet, professor of medicine and chief of nephrology in the Faculté de Médecine in Paris, generously provided access to those of his grandfather's documents that are in his possession. At Charles' death his library and his personal effects were pretty well dispersed. He left his collection of theses to the Société de Biologie and his physiology books to the laboratory of physiology at the Faculté de Médecine in Paris. Other books, including those on social science and physical science, he willed to the Institut Marey located in Paul Bert's former laboratory in the Bois de Boulogne. His remaining books and personal effects were supposed to have been divided among his remaining children. Gabriel tried hard to collect or obtain photocopies of his grandfather's documents that had been scattered among family members. Unfortunately he found that many had been lost. Sadly, he was unable to find any trace of notebooks that contained the original records of his grandfather's experimental work.

During August 1986, Gabriel and his wife Claude generously welcomed me into their summer home in the hills of Provence. For nearly a week they allowed me to study and photograph the materials that they had on hand. Particularly helpful was a five volume, 1500-page diary-style memoir written by Charles Richet during World War I, mainly in 1916, with additions in subsequent years. With the title *Mémoires sur moi et les autres*, it was intended for his children and grandchildren so that, as he put it, "they would know the full truth of my life and my accomplishments. I can't tell everything: Any man who says he does is lying."

In the *Mémoires* Richet expressed his wish that it be kept private for his children and grandchildren for several years but he gave the right of publication to his grandson, Charles, the son of his oldest child, George, "if he is able to find an editor." Charles died at age eighty-two. Another of the older grandsons, Gabriel, who continues in excellent health, has authorized me to make certain references to the *Mémoires*, but does not want it to be published or freely quoted.

My reading was supplemented by lengthy recorded interviews with Gabriel. He knew his grandfather well and spoke freely and frankly about him, about some of his associates and students, about university politics and about the views and comments of some of his grandfather's colleagues.

Following my visit, Gabriel continued to provide help by checking and filling in countless details in the manuscript. I am deeply in his debt.

After leaving Provence I went to Paris where Professor Michel Conte, recently retired as professor in the Faculté de Médecine at Paris helped me greatly in locating material in the library of the old Faculté de Médecine where Richet had worked and in identifying and photographing Richet's various homes and laboratories that were scattered around Paris.

Next I journeyed to the Mediterranean coast of France and visited the Château Richet at Carqueiranne, purchased in 1872 by Charles' father, Alfred. I identified Charles' former research aquarium, now a swimming club, and visited the beautiful Ile Ribaud where Gabriel's daughter, Marie Claude and her family were vacationing. I am grateful to them for enabling me to see firsthand and to photograph a place that was very significant in the life of Charles Richet.

Professor André Cournand, who had been a student at the medical school in Paris when Richet was still teaching, provided many helpful reminiscences and introduced me to some of the "old timers" who had known Richet and who still held important positions in French medical science.

In late spring and early summer of 1988 I returned to Paris where again Gabriel Richet helped with further inquiries. I also visited and interviewed Charles Richet's only surviving son, Alfred Richet. At age ninety-five he was alert, engaging and immensely cooperative in answering questions and providing reminiscences. Both he and his son, Denis, to whom he introduced me emphasized Charles Richet's unfettered individuality and courage in defending his own convictions. Denis was immensely helpful in furnishing me with copies of important family documents. He died suddenly in September 1989.

Mme. France Montebello de Baecque, the granddaughter of Richet's cousin Madeleine, whom he deeply loved, gave me a picture of her grandmother as a young woman, a letter to Richet from her mother, and a privately printed book, *L'Isle Adam*, written by Mme. de Baecque, that included the history of her family's country home, the château de Stors, and its surroundings.

I also visited the château Villandry near Tours, which had been purchased in 1906 by Anna Coleman and Joachim Carvallo, a couple who had worked in Richet's laboratory and to both of whom he had been very close. I talked with the present owner, Joachim's grandson, Robert, who gave me several documents concerning his grandfather and grandmother including their photographs and copies of letters they had received from Charles Richet. I am deeply grateful to all of the above relatives and friends of Charles Richet who have helped fill in and verify the details of his life.

A much revered former teacher of mine at Johns Hopkins Medical School and a world renowned scholar in medical history, Dr. Saul Jarcho, carefully reviewed the manuscript at various stages and offered valuable advice and guidance. Help with writing style and clarity was provided by the accomplished author William Davenport. Dr. Frederick L. Holmes, professor and chairman of the Department of the History of Medicine at Yale University, an authority on Richet, has generously and patiently served as the principal consultant for this work.

I am also indebted to my son George Wolf for scholarly advice, to Professors Charles Rosenberg, Gert Brieger, and Diana Long, medical historians who made helpful criticisms and suggestions for shaping the text, to Helen Goodell for her assistance in the preparation of this manuscript, to Maria Collette for bibliographic searches, to Barbara Griffin for assistance with study in various libraries in the U.S., and to Judith Jones and Betty Ball for typing and retyping the revisions, and especially to Joy A. Lowe for her patient and skillful assistance throughout the development of the manuscript.

Irving Louis Horowitz, president and Mary Curtis, publisher of Transaction Publishers have taken a special interest in the Richet manuscript. I am grateful to them for facilitating its publication and to Esther Luckett for skillfully implementing its production.

A grant from the Eleanor Naylor Dana Charitable Trust made the work possible. My deep appreciation goes to the Trust and its Board of Trustees.

Richet Chronology

1850	Birth.
1861	Entered Lycée.
	Wrote poems and plays.
	Published *Maximes de la vie*.
1864	Death of paternal grandmother.
1866	Hypnotized young friend of his sister.
1867	Graduated from Lycée and passed baccalaureate to study medicine and science.
1868	Entered University.
1870	Franco-Prussian War.
	Service as Guard at Invalides.
1872	Rotating intern service.
	Father bought château at Carqueiranne.
1873	Internship with surgeon Lefort.
	Decision to become a physiologist.
1874	Work in laboratory of Marey.
	Began study of crayfish muscle.
	Published *La suggestion mentale et le Calcul des probabilités*.
1875	Published *Le Somnambulisme Provoqué*.
1876	Internship with Verneuil.
	Work in lab of Berthelot.
	Study of gastric sensation and gastric juice in Marcellin.
	Published *De l'état fontionnel des nerfs dans l'hemianesthésie hystérique*.
1877	M.D. thesis.
	Published *Recherches Expérimentales et Cliniques sur la Sensibilité*.

1878   Sc.D. thesis. Death of maternal grandfather.
            Appointed Agrégé. Marriage. Back to Marey's lab
            and started in Vulpian's lab. Published *Du suc
            Gastrique chez l'homme et les Animaux*. Discovery
            of "fast" and "slow" muscles, the phenomena of
            refractory period and summation in nerves and
            demonstrated summation in vision with Antoine
            Breguet. Studies on nervous control of heartbeat.
            Published *Structure des circonvolutions cérébrales*.

1879   Discovered diuretic effect of sugars. Completed
            translation of *De Motu Cordis* by William Harvey.

1880   Published *Contribution à la physiologie des centres
            nerveux et des muscles de l'écrevisse*. Began study
            of anesthetics and poisons.

1881   Editor of *Revue Scientifique*. Continued study of
            hypnosis. Wrote *A la Recherche de la Gloire, Une
            Conscience d'homme* and others including
            Pierrot Vendu.

1882   Published *Physiologie des Muscles et des Nerfs*. Studies
            of digestion in fish.

1883   Began studies of thermoregulatory mechanisms.
            Discovered heat loss in dogs by panting. Published
            La personnalité et la mémoire dans le somnambulism.

1884   Joined Société de la Paix. Built siphon calorimeter.
            Discovered the cerebral trigger for fever and
            published *La fièvre traumatique nerveuse et
            L'influence des lésions de cerveau sur la
            température générale*. Published *Lavoisier et la
            chaleur animale* and *Man's right over animals*.

1885   Published *Recherches de calorimetrie*. Published *Essai
            de psycholgoie générale*.
            Death of mother.

1886   Published *De l'action physiologique des sels alcalins;
            études de toxicologie générale*. Elected to the
            Society for Psychical Research.

1887   Purchase of le Ribaud. Appointed professor of
        physiology. Retirement of father.
        Elected to Society for Psychical Research (UK).
        Discovered the brain's role in body temperature
        regulation. Metabolic experiments with Hanriot.
        First experiments on passive immunity. Published
        *Leçons sur la chaleur animale; la respiration et la
        temperature.* Experience with psychics. Visit to Milan.
        Published *Possession, L'homme et l'Intelligence.*

1888   Start development of aircraft with Tatin. Published
        *Sur un microbe pyogène et septique (Staphylyococcus
        pyrosepticus) et sur la vaccination contre ses
        effets.* Disappointing efforts to immunize against TB.

1889   Eiffel Tower meeting of psychologists and philosophers.
        Studies of starvation. Published *Cécité psychique
        experimentale chez le chien.*

1890   Founded "Annales des Sciences Psychiques." First
        administration of "serotherapy" to a patient.
        Published further experiments in hypnotic lucidity
        or clairvoyance.

1891   Death of father. Published *Pour les grands et les
        petits, fables.*

1892   Zomotherapy.

1893   Discovery of Chloralose. Work on arbitration among
        nations.

1894   The dive reflex effect of asphyxia on heart rate.
        Published *Bibliographia Physiologica.*

1895   Published *Dictionnaire de Physiologie.*

1896   Further studies on pain. Early study of anorexia nervosa.

1897   Published *Periode réfractaire dans les centres nerveux*
        with Broca. Published biographical note.

1898   President Société de Biologie; Elected to Académie de
        Médecine. Published *Histoire Universel des Nations;
        Soeur Marthe* as a play.

1899   Published *La résistance des canards à l'asphyxie.*
        Published *Les guerre et la paix: Etude sur l'arbitrage
        international.*

1900   President of World Congress of Peace in Paris.

1901   Published Note *sur un cas remarquable de précocité
        musicale.*

1902   First experiment on anaphylaxis; published *De l'action
        anaphylactique de certains venins.* Completed *Circé.*

1903   The use of bromides with low chloride diet in epilepsy.
        Published *Etude sur un cas de prémonition.*

1904   Published *Death of Socrates.*

1905   President of Society for Psychical Research (UK); Several
        publications on metapsychology. Performance of
        Circé with Sarah Bernhardt at Théatre de Monte Carlo.

1906   More publications on metapsychology.

1907   Published *Le passé de la querre et l'avenir de la paix.*

1908   Published *The pros and cons of Vivisection.* Published *An
        enquiry into premonitions.*

1909   Passive transfer of anaphylaxis predicted; Published
        *Role du Système Nerveux dans les Phénomènes de le
        anaphylaxie.*

1910   Predicted neurotransmitters in lecture to International
        Congress of Physiologists; Published *L'humorisme
        ancien et l'humorisme moderne discours prononcé
        au congrès de physiologie.*

1911   Published *L'anaphylaxie.*

1912   Prix de Moscou. Twenty-five Year Festschrift. Published
        Histoire Générale.

1913   Nobel Prize.

1914   Elected to Académie des Sciences; poetry prize by
        Académie Française; War work, trips to Italy,
        Russia. Published *La Gloire de Pasteur*; and
        autobiographical note.

1916   Death of son-in-law in combat. Published *Les évènements psychiques de la guerre. Un appel de M. Charles Richet aux soldats; avez-vous des pressentiments?* Published *Les Coupables.*

1917   Prevention of surgical shock in wounded soldiers with chloralose.German publication of *Histoire Générale.*

1918   Performed plasma transfusions at front in WWI after preliminary experiments on haemorrhagic shock in animals.Son, Albert, shot down and killed.Croix de Guerre. Working for peace.

1919   Published *L'anesthésie dans les blessures de guerre.* Published *L'homme stupide; La selection humaine* and French edition *Abrégé d'histoire générale.*

1921   Published *Traité de physiologie médico chirurgicale with Charles fils.* Published *Les ténèbres de l'heure.*

1922   Published *Traité de métapsychique.*

1923   Published Dictionnaire de Physiologie; vol. 10; *Le Savant.*

1924   Published *La Nouvelle Zomotherapie.*

1925   Retirement as professor

1926   Grand Officier de la Légion d'honneur. Festschrift at Académie de Médecine. Published *Aux jeunes gens des écoles de tous les pays. Histoire universelle des civilisations.*

1927   Published *Notre Sixième Sens.*

1930   Published *L'age d'or et l'age de l'or.*

1931   Published *L'avenir et la prémonition.*

1932   President of Académie des Sciences. Short autobiography.

1933   Published *La Grande Espérance.*

1934   Published *Souvenirs d'un Physiologiste.*

1935   Published *Au Seuil de la Mystère; Au Secours.* Death.

1

Charles Richet's Background and the Shaping of His Endeavor 1850–1869

Richet—*c'est un nom de Seigneur*, a lordly name, as they say in France. The most widely known and clearly the most lordly bearer of that name was Charles Richet, professor of physiology at the Faculté de Médecine in Paris from 1887 to 1925.

There were other distinguished medical Richets: father Alfred, who held the chair in surgery in the Faculté de Médecine and served as chief surgeon at the Hôtel Dieu, the post formerly held by the famous surgeon Guillaume Dupuytren (1777–1835), Charles' son, Charles *fils*, who became professor of medicine and grandson, Gabriel, professor of medicine, recently retired. The Richet dynasty held full professorships at the Faculté de Médecine of Paris during 122 years from 1864 to 1986.

Charles Richet is best known for the discovery of anaphylaxis that, from studies begun in 1902, won him the Nobel Prize in 1913. Anaphylaxis is a severe and potentially fatal hypersensitivity reaction induced by an injection of a foreign substance, usually a protein, to which an individual has already been sensitized. Richet devised the term from the Greek *ana* and *phylaxis*, meaning "against protection," to contrast with the word prophylaxis, meaning "for protection."

Richet's discoveries, made while exploring the phenomena of anaphylaxis, actually linked hypersensitivity to protection and thereby led to the unraveling of the mystery of immunity conferred by vaccination and inoculation. They led ultimately to our current understanding of the role of the nerves in regulating the immune system. In this and others of his discoveries Richet's primary contribution was conceptual, the concept being that the manifestations of disease constitute the body's own protective response to invaders rather than representing incursive damage done by external forces. Further, on the basis of evidence adduced by

1

Richet, the concept holds that the body's adaptive efforts to protect against or contain agents of disease are instituted and regulated in the brain. Richet's central concern was the protection and perfecting of the human organism, an intellectual agenda so broad that most of his physiological contributions, although often original, were fragmentary. His curious mind was subject to distraction by a wide range of concerns including some outside the range of physiology that in his view related, nevertheless, to the objective of enhancing the quality of the human race.

The promise of eugenics was one such concern that held great appeal for Richet and he devoted much time to it. In a monograph distributed in manuscript form to some of his colleagues and ultimately published in 1919, Richet wrote, "nothing is more extraordinary than our indifference to human selection. One could laugh if it were not so unfortunate. We improve breeds of chickens, ducks, horses, pigs, lambs, even species of cauliflower, beets, strawberries, and violets! Man improves and perfects everything except man himself."[R 595] Richet favored limiting procreation by the deformed and the intellectually handicapped, but encouraged large families for those potentially able to contribute to civilization.

Interest in eugenics grew out of the work of Charles Darwin (1809–1882) that had great appeal for Richet although most French biologists at the time were skeptical of Darwin's book, *Origin of Species* (Darwin 1859), belittled it, or were openly antagonistic. Others credited Darwin only with having extended or refined the work of Jean Baptiste Pierre Antoine de Monet, Chevalier de Lamarck (1744–1829). Even Richet, in his book *Physiologie des Muscles et des Nerfs*, wrote that the theory of evolution was "conceived by Lamarck and Etienne Geoffrey St. Hilaire (1772–1844), our two illustrious compatriots; it was revived, recreated afresh, so to speak, and popularized by Charles Darwin."[R 98]

Richet was also concerned with the loss to France of fine human specimens in wars. Richet opposed war and considered pacifism the best way to preserve the world's human potential, especially that of France.

Another area, seemingly peripheral to physiology, but one that Richet viewed as potentially useful toward the full development of humanity and in which he made a large personal investment, was an aspect of

Citations for Richet's publications are indicated by the letter R followed by the numerical listing in the Richet bibliography. Quotations from unpublished notes and interviews with family members are given the citation (Unp). Titles of publications, mainly novels and plays not located or identified, are given the citation (Nid).

spiritualism for which he coined the term "metapsychique." He saw extrasensory perception as a physiological capability that had not been fully developed and should therefore become the object of serious scientific study.

Finally, as a way of elevating the human species, Richet turned to the humanities, history philosophy and literature, both prose and poetry. His poetry twice won special recognition from the Académie Française. Literature was for Richet a means of growth and a respite from daily demands and responsibilities. It separated him from outside influences, thus allowing full play to his thoughts and imagination. As Richet himself put it "by living in the world of men one ends perforce by losing one's identity. As one's differentiating originality disappears, one ceases to think for oneself for the sake of thinking like others, which is equivalent to no longer thinking at all . . . [of] an indisputably higher order than the activity of doing . . . is the activity of dreaming" (Nock 1934).

There were other European scientists who contributed serious literary works including the distinguished physiologists, Albrecht von Haller (1708-1777), Claude Bernard (1813-1878), and Charles Jules Henri Nicolle (1866-1936), for example, and several took political posts in the French government on the side, but none spread his interests and activities so broadly as did Richet. His curiosity was boundless, as was his desire to excel in each of his endeavors, but he shifted from one to another at his whim as each seemed important to his goal of human improvement. Except for his study of anaphylaxis and two or three others of his physiological studies Richet failed to fully exploit his talents in either science or literature and thoroughly "wrap up" an undertaking. Nevertheless, Richet's seemingly diffuse approach to problems in physiology yielded him shrewd and subtle perceptions from which he formulated a unifying concept of health and disease based on adaptation, genetic, physiological and behavioral. As his colleague, Emile Gley (1857-1930) expressed it, "He sees the major functions of the organism as mechanisms of defense." (Gley 1926). Richet's clearly purposeful surmise was closely akin to a more recent formulation by H.G. Wolff (1899-1962) who viewed diseases as protective adaptive patterns elicited in response to all manner of assaults, tangible and intangible (Wolff 1953).

Background and Early Development

This multifaceted man who felt a need to improve the world was born to privilege at his parents home 11 rue Louis le Grand in Paris on 25 August 1850. His affluent parents enjoyed a high social position. His father, formal and austere, was driven by a single purpose, to excel as an academic surgeon. His mother, quiet and correct, was a deeply religious Roman Catholic. Young Charles was perhaps more attached to his maternal grandparents than to his parents.

Every Thursday and Sunday there were family dinners at the home of his maternal grandparents, the Renouards, on the rue de Provence. Young Charles was given the special privilege of sitting with the men after dinner as his grandfather and uncle Alfred Renouard smoked their pipes and father Alfred, his cigar. Richet's first favorite among the books in his grandfather's large library was the *Fables de La Fontaine*, but Charles Renouard (1794–1878), who often read to his grandson in Latin, eventually aroused his interest in the classics. As he grew older, Charles not only adopted many of his grandfather's literary tastes, but his love of the sea and his philosophical views and values as well, especially his democratic convictions and his hatred of war and Napoleon. Richet's quick mind and beguiling manners made him the favorite of his grandmother as well as his grandfather whom he idolized and from whom he acquired his interest in sailing and his love for Latin and classical literature.

Family Connections

The influence of Richet's father in the medical faculty gave a powerful boost to his son's academic ambitions. Beyond that, the prominence of his relatives and forebears was an important asset in enabling him, at a young age, to become an editor of two widely read journals and to operate in a broad arena, moving back and forth from science to humanities.

Richet's maternal great grandfather, Antoine Auguste Renouard (1765–1854), a manufacturer of gauze and later a full time bibliophile and publisher, had been a prominent figure in Paris during the Convention. Married to the illegitimate daughter of the Marquis de Beauchamp, he had worked successfully for the preservation of precious art objects and books and managed to save many of them from the mass destruction carried out during the violence of the revolution. Richet's grandfather, Charles Renouard, had himself participated in the strategy for the Revolution of 1830 that overthrew the Bourbon King Charles X. A liberal journalist and specialist in admiralty law, he hated Napoleon. When at age sixteen his performance in the "Concours General," a competitive examination given to the upperclassmen at the Lycées, earned him an appointment [scholarship] to the Sorbonne, he refused it because the successful candidate was required to give a eulogy of Napoleon's son, the King of Rome.

Charles Renouard married Adèle Girard, the daughter of a wealthy engineer, Pierre Simon Girard (1765-1836), who was born in Caen into a family of strict Calvinist watchmakers.

A brilliant student, especially in mathematics, Pierre Simon, in 1790, won a prize in engineering offered by the Académie des Sciences. His capabilities were recognized by General Bonaparte, soon to become the Emperor Napoleon. Bonaparte took him along as commander of the brigade of engineers on his conquest of Egypt. Napoleon, with his characteristically patronizing attitude toward other nations, intended to rescue the Egyptians from their ignorance and brutality by exposing them to the intellectual riches of France. At the same time he wanted their ancient civilization to be studied and their arts, literature, science, and architecture to be brought to the attention of the French. He succeeded in establishing the Institut d'Egypte, modeled after the French Academies, but he was more successful in recruiting scientists and engineers for the project than musicians, poets, and artists. In the party with Girard were the chemist Claude Louis Bertholet (1748-1822) the mathematicians Gaspard Monge (1746-1818), Jean Baptiste Joseph Fourier (1768-1830), and the naturalist, Etienne Geoffroy Saint Hilaire who did early work in embryology. The Institut, established in a place close to Cairo, contained printing presses for both Arabic and Latin types, laboratories for chemistry and physics and a library. Girard was not only a founding member of the Institute d'Egypte but he also became Bonaparte's minister of the Interior of Egypt. His task was to develop a plan for a canal at Suez and to establish a great port on the Red Sea athwart the shipping route to the Indies as a challenge to Great Britain.[1] After his return to France he was offered an important political post by the future emperor Napoleon. Girard declined, however, and elected to continue as an engineer.

With Napoleon's support he built a canal from a tributary of the Marne to the Seine at Paris, the Canal de l'Ourcq. Largely for this accomplishment he was elected to membership in the Institut de France. Since the Renouard family were strict Roman Catholics and the Girards were not at all religious, Girard's daughter Adèle had to take her first communion shortly before her marriage to Charles Renouard. It was their daughter, Eugénie, who married Alfred Richet in 1849.

Charles Richet's paternal forebears were less socially and politically prominent. His great grandfather, Gaspard Richet (1737-1819), was a descendent of a long line of master locksmiths who had lived for four generations in Burgundy in the vicinity of Dijon. The family had migrated from Champagne where Richet is still a common name. There are also many Richets in Normandy. In 1810 Gaspard's son, François, at age sixty married as his second wife Victoire Choffez, the daughter of an innkeeper in Luxeuil who had sent her to Dijon to apprentice to a milliner. Charles Richet's father, Didier Dominique Alfred, born in 1816, was the youngest of two surviving children of François and Victoire. When Alfred was three years old his father died, leaving Victoire barely able to support her children on the income of her millinery shop. Young Alfred had acquired an interest in medicine from a maternal uncle named Lombard, a Navy surgeon who lived near Dijon.[2] His father Claude-Antoine Lombard (1741-1811) was well known as professor of surgery at l'Ecole de Service de Santé Militaire in Strasbourg under Louis XVI.

Victoire, recognizing the precociousness in her son Alfred, sent him to Paris at age eighteen with a bottle of Dijon Cassis and a monthly allowance of sixty francs. Alfred did well in medical school, achieved the highest grades and, on graduation in 1839, competed successfully for an internship in the Paris hospitals. He further pursued his education in medicine under the tutelage of the famous surgeon Alfred Louis Armand Marie Velpeau (1795-1867). Shortly after graduation from medical school he published original studies on vascular tumors of bone for which he was awarded the "Grand Prix" of the Académie des Sciences in 1851 (Richet, A. 1864). Eager to earn an appointment as Agrégé, faculty associate at the University of Paris, but having limited financial resources, he had to spend most of each day in surgical practice.[3] Evenings were devoted to writing a book on surgical anatomy. Finally published in 1855, his *Traité Pratique d'Anatomie Chirurgicale* was the culmination of long sustained effort. The first edition was so well received that a second edition was required within two years (Richet, A. 1855-57). This important book remained a standard authority on the subject for fifty years. In 1864 Alfred was appointed professor of surgery at the Faculté de Médecine in Paris. In 1865 he was elected to the Académie de Médecine and eventually to the Académie des Sciences. Alfred and Eugénie Renouard married in 1849. The following year Charles Richet was born and two years later his sister, Louise. Richet's parents and grandparents shared the pattern of upward mobility typical of the age, as the *petits bourgeois* became *grands bourgeois* and rose to become the social leaders.

Charles Richet was named for his grandfather, Charles Renouard. His middle name, Robert, was for his father's close friend, Robert Bazille. Bazille's wife, Rose, had grown up in the same pension as Adèle Renouard. It was through the Bazilles that Alfred and his wife Eugénie had met.

One day when Mme. Bazille, who was very short, visited his mother, young Charles called out loudly, "Mamma, is she a dwarf?" Later, he wrote in his *Mémoires*: "What an ingrate, a triple ingrate, I was. When she died in 1872 she left me, her husband's namesake, 2000 francs to be contributed to a 'good cause.' I gave it to L'Association d'Alsace Lorraine" (Unp).

Despite his effrontery, the little boy quickly became the favorite of his grandmother Adèle who, he acknowledged, indulged him and openly favored him over her other grandchildren.

Growing Up

When he was in the fifth grade Charles' mother, a devout Catholic, took him to the church of St. Louis d'Antin for his first communion administered by the Abbé Caron. Impressed by that experience, Charles promised the abbé to become a priest although it appeared to him that neither his father nor grandfather had manifested much interest in the church. His mother told young Charles that his father attended mass at the hospital. Charles believed her for a time until his inevitable discovery of the truth and his disillusionment. Grandfather Renouard attended mass but did not go to confession or take communion. Soon Charles himself began to doubt ecclesiastical dogmas and to question the authority of the church. He eventually became a confirmed agnostic. In his *Mémoires* he wrote that he "had long and painful anguish" as he gradually abandoned the faith of his childhood. Although he expressed tenderness toward his mother, he made little mention of family activities or his relationship with his father.

In sharp contrast to his father's early pattern of life, Charles' youthful years were very little devoted to study. Instead, with his cousin Robert Girard and his school friends, he enjoyed parties, plays, boating, fishing, card games, travel and gambling at Monte Carlo (Unp). At home indoors their favorite game was whist until Richet and his friend Emile Bardier invented a new but similar game, Gobefiche, that they considered even more fun. Richet was also enthusiastic about bridge which he continued to play until his death.

Father Alfred found his relaxation and enjoyment in the countryside where he operated with deep interest as a gentleman farmer. Charles, on the other hand, like his grandfather Renouard, loved the sea and had little interest in crops or flowers: "without doubt" he wrote "it is because I lacked patience; it takes too long to grow them" (Unp). Charles did enjoy hunting on his father's large farm at Lépine in Brie near Mormant (Seine et Marne), but after his father's death in 1891, he gave up hunting because, as he wrote, "the train ride seemed to provoke severe head-aches."

Richet's autobiographical writings contain no account of contacts with his paternal grandparents. In fact his grandfather François Richet had died long before his birth and he saw his paternal grandmother Victoire only once before she died in 1864. He did, however, see a good deal of his father's older sister Herminie who lived in Paris with her husband, Auguste Voisin, an alcoholic ne'er-do-well and womanizer. Charles was very solicitous of their daughter, Bertha, who married a cold and also unfaithful husband.

In 1861 Charles' father moved the family to 8 rue Drouout in the ninth arrondissement. From there young Charles attended the Lycée Bona-parte.[4] At the Lycée Charles had applied himself very little to his studies except for Latin and literature. He especially disliked mathematics. He spent much of his time writing poetry and plays. With his friend Paul Fournier he wrote a book of verses, Le Livre d'Or de la Comtesse Diane, containing games and "bon mots" that were eventually published as Maximes de la Vie (Nid). Charles and a close friend of his sister, Amélie Demarest, often performed his plays for family and friends at the Demarest house. His favorite was *Maitre Guerin*. On reconsidering it later in life, however, he judged it "quite mediocre" (Unp).

Richet's maternal grandmother, Adèle, impressed by his literary abilities, had not wanted him to study medicine, but his father clearly had tried to interest him in the field. While he was still at the Lycée, Alfred had taken Charles to the Hôtel Dieu to see "a rare operation"—a blood transfusion. Richet wrote in his *Souvenirs d'un Physiologiste* that he had studied medicine largely because he thought it would please his father.[R736]

In 1869, after Charles' graduation from the Lycée the family moved to 25 Boulevard Haussmann. He passed his baccalaureate examinations "without a single day of preparation," as he expressed it, making him eligible to study medicine and also to take a science degree (Unp).

Richet, clearly nurtured by the times, emerged as passionately dedicated to individual independence and freedom from regimentation. His political convictions were democratic, but, like his grandfather and great grandfather Renouard, his social tastes and behavior were aristocratic. Having rejected religion, he adopted instead the biological dogma, generally attributed to Charles Darwin, that only the fittest deserve to survive. Perhaps consistent with such a self-centered view, Richet was also attracted to the opulent self-indulgence of the "ancien régime" as it was echoed in the voluptuous atmosphere of the Second Empire that prevailed during Charles' youth. His life also reflected the energy, intensity, and restlessness of the period. He enjoyed the works of Pascal, Bossuet, Musset, and Flaubert but he considered Corneille tiresome and was totally opposed to the writings of Jean Jacques Rousseau (1712–1778) (Unp.).

According to his grandson, Gabriel, Charles Richet had very little interest in the graphic arts and music[5] although the taste for innovation characteristic of the contemporary artists and composers, their defiance of current dogmas, their sacrifice of detail for feeling and for elegance of execution were thoroughly consonant with Richet's proclivities. His dedication to challenging traditional dogma, his championship of the "offbeat," his involvement in causes and his appetite for innovation certainly fitted the mood of the impressionist painters. Like them he sought for a quick perception of nature and a quick but penetrating rendition of his interpretations. Perhaps Renoir, who blended elegance with sharp-eyed simplicity and directness was, among the impressionist painters, the closest match to Richet. Many of the artists, Renoir among them, who today are considered the most distinguished of their time, were never elected to the Académie des Beaux Arts. Richet, too, had had difficulty with acceptance by the intellectual arbiters of his day. He was turned down four times for election to the Académie des Sciences and was admitted only after he won the Nobel Prize. He applied twice to the Académie Française but was rebuffed each time, despite his work having been twice honored by the Académie itself.

Notes

1. The idea of a canal had been discussed and several times attempted since the time of the Pharaoh of Egypt. An inscription on the temple at Karnak refers to such a canal in the time of Seti (1380 B.C.). In more recent times Gotfried Wilhelm Baron Von Leibniz (1646–1716) had suggested to Louis XIV that he construct such a canal but the king declined. The isthmus was surveyed at Napoleon's request by the engineer Lepère but, because he erroneously concluded that there was approximately a thirty foot difference between the sea level of the Red Sea and the Mediterranean, the idea was abandoned.
2. Lombard was captured with his ship by pirates in 1803. The crew were taken as prisoners to Tunis and put in the galleys. Lombard, however, became the court physician of the Bey of Tunis and also his prisoner. In 1818 the Bey allowed him to visit France on his promise to return. Despite his promise, Lombard remained in France.
3. There were no full-time clinical faculty members in those days. Most of the medical faculty earned a living through practice.
4. Now known as the Lycée Condorcet.
5. About chamber music Richet wrote in his *Mémoires*: "Do you know why people applaud? Because it is over."

2

Postrevolutionary Developments That Influenced Richet and His Work

The political situation that prevailed at the time of Charles Richet's birth was described by Alexis de Tocqueville (1805–1859) in his *Recollections* (Mayer 1948). Tocqueville's notes, made between 1848 and 1850, provide a vivid and perceptive insight into the political crosscurrents and the international deals that were designed to keep France afloat and in which he, himself, as minister of foreign affairs, had played a major role. The Revolution of 1848 led to the fall of the constitutional monarchy under Louis Philippe. A republic was reestablished but, as de Tocqueville noted, the French were still unable to shake off their need for the central authority. He doubted the wisdom of universal suffrage by a largely uninformed populace accustomed to autocratic rule. "The republican form of government" he wrote, "is not the best suited to the needs of France . . . government without checks always promises more, but gives less liberty than a constitutional monarchy"[1] (Mayer 1948).

Despite de Tocqueville's warning the people opted for a republic. Four years later, however, his judgment was vindicated as the elected president, Louis Napoleon, was awarded his uncle's mantle as emperor by the coup d'etat of 1852.

From the swirling maelstrom of postrevolutionary ideas and aspirations, the bourgeois class emerged to dominate the social and political structure of France. Many of the technocrats, scientists, writers, and artists from bourgeois families became involved in politics, government, and administration where they presided over rapidly fluctuating social prescriptions.

If there was a unifying theme in the chaotic and conflicting social and intellectual developments in postrevolutionary France, it was resistance to regimentation and distrust of restraints imposed by traditional author-

11

ity. The intellectual and emotional rebellion of the French people found
common ground in opposition to the papacy and the power of its clerics.
Not surprisingly among many, including the distinguished historian-phi-
losopher Ernest Renan (1823–1892) who had started his career as a
Catholic seminarist, the anticlerical attitude was translated into a more
general rejection of religion. Various ethical philosophies were proposed
as substitutes for traditional Christianity. Through the cacophony of
voices and the confusion of competing ideas, the goal of personal liberty
was shared among the various factions, but their views as to how to
achieve the common goal differed radically.

Arts and Letters

The changes in French political emphasis were matched by equally
radical shifts in artistic expression. The main literary currents in Nineteenth-century France are usually characterized, somewhat artificially,
as romanticism, referring to the work of Larmartine and Hugo, realism
as exemplified by Balzac and Zola, and symbolism, expressed most
vividly by the work of Baudelaire. The edges of these classifications are
blurred and the emphases put forward in the work of a single author were
often contradictory. Ernest Renan, a member of the Académie Française
embodied the versatility and the shifting allegiances of French intellectual leaders. Renan was something of an arbiter among those seeking
admission to the Académie Française and to the Académie des Sciences
Morale et Politique as well. Richet's interests, beliefs and behavior
mirrored many of those of Renan. Renan, although deeply interested in
science, was also a poet of delicate sensitivity. Having grown up as a
pious rationalist, he propounded a positivist point of view in his *Life of
Jesus* denying the divinity of Christ (Renan 1863). Renan characterized
himself as "a romantic protesting against romanticism, a Utopian preach-
ing the practical a tissue of contradictions." "And yet," he added "it has
brought me the most lively intellectual enjoyment one could savor"
(quoted in Lagarde 1955). Thus the contradictions of nineteenth-century
France were coupled with a remarkable ebullience and an inclination
toward experimentation and change.

The trend toward innovation was especially evident in the graphic arts
during Richet's youth. Although he had little interest in painting, his taste
for elegance, for surprise, and for freedom seems to have reflected the

spirit of the romantic forerunners of the impressionist painters, Eugène Delacroix (1798-1865) in particular. Delacroix's paintings had won praise during the 1820s at the salons sponsored by the Académie des Beaux Arts. Soon, however, he became deeply influenced by the work of the English innovators, William Blake (1757-1857), Joseph Mallord Turner (1775-1851), and especially by John Constable (1776-1837) whose paintings were shown at the Paris Salon of 1824 and whom Delacroix praised as "one of the glories of England." Delacroix's subsequent magnificent but unorthodox freedom with subject, form, color, and light delayed his election to the Académie for thirty years.

The French Government During and After the Revolution

1789 - 1791	Social and Land Reforms under Louis XVI
1791 - 1795	Abolition of Royalty - The Turbulent Bourgeois
1795 - 1799	The Directoire
1799 - 1804	The Consulate (Abbé Sieyes, Roger-Ducos, Bonaparte)
1804 - 1814	The Empire (Napoleon I)
1815 - 1824	Louis XVIII
1824 - 1830	Charles X
1830 - 1848	Louis Philippe
1848 - 1852	Revolution and Second Republic (Louis-Napoleon)
1852 - 1870	Second Empire (Napoleon III)
1870 - 1940	Third Republic, briefly interrupted by the commune, 1871

The Academies

Among the powerful voices in nineteenth-century Paris were those of the members of the Institut de France, comprised of the elite Academies. The Académie Française, designed to promote and oversee literary and artistic matters, had been established in 1635 under the patronage of Cardinal Richelieu during the reign of Louis XIII. Previously the literati had gathered regularly at the house of the king's secretary, Valentin

Courart. The Académie des Sciences, which had been organized by René Descartes (1596-1650), Pierre Gassendi (1592-1655), Blaise Pascal (1623-1662), and his father Etienne (1588-1651), was given the official sanction of the state by Louis XIV in 1666.[2]

The membership of the Académie des Sciences included several foreign scientists of distinction. Its proceedings were recorded in Latin by the permanent secretary. The first of these was Jean Baptiste Duhamel (1624-1706). During the French Revolution the people's hatred of aristocratic rank and privilege extended to the aristocracy of learning as exemplified by the Academies. Accordingly they were abolished in 1793 by the Convention and some of their members, including Antoine Laurent Lavoisier (1743-1794) were guillotined. In 1795 the Directoire revived them as the Institut National des Sciences et des Arts. In 1800, Bonaparte, now premier consul of France, was elected president of the Institut. Later, in 1816, Louis XVIII revived the title, Academy. Ultimately the Académie des Sciences and the other academies dedicated to fine arts, inscriptions, and moral and political sciences also regained their names as units of the Institut with the Académie Française, committed to literature and the protection of the French language, ranked superior to the others.

The Spread of Experimental Physiology from Italy to Germany to France

The roots of experimental physiology extend at least as far back as Andrea Cesalpino (1519-1603), Italian physician and botanist who, with experiments using venous ligation, identified the circulation of the blood fifty years before William Harvey (1578-1657) in Great Britain published his beautifully designed experiments in 1628. (Harvey 1628). In Italy, Giovanni Alphonso Borelli (1608-1679), in the tradition of Harvey's contemporary Galileo Galilei (1564-1642), applied physics to the study of the functions of the human body (Borelli 1680). Borelli's work was carried further by Marcello Malpighi (1628-1694) who brought the newly invented microscope into play. With it he confirmed Harvey's assumption concerning the passage of blood through the lungs by demonstrating, microscopically, the pulmonary capillaries (Malpighi 1661). He also confirmed Borelli's predictions that within tissues of the animal body would be found small structures that provide the means of mechanical and chemical work (Malpighi 1661). Another Italian, Luigi Galvani (1737-1798), made a major contribution to physiology with the brilliant discovery that electricity was involved in natural muscular movement (Galvani 1981).

By the nineteenth-century the leadership in experimental physiology had shifted from Italy to Germany where Johannes Müller (1801-1858) who, by applying the principles of physics in his experiments, enhanced current understanding of color vision and voice production (Müller 1834). Julius Robert Von Mayer (1814-1878), showed that the physical law of the conservation of energy was operative in living beings (Von Mayer 1842). Herman Von Helmholtz (1821-1894) was, perhaps, the greatest of the German physiologists. Among his many original contributions was the measurement of the velocity of electrical conduction in nerves. His wide interests and accomplishments in neurophysiology encompassed psychology as well. Carl Ludwig (1816-1895), under whom Richet's teacher, Etienne Jules Marey (1830-1904) studied, was responsible for several important methodologic contributions including the kymograph, a device for graphic recording during animal experimentation.

In France physiology was being taught by and under the control of anatomists and surgeons, among them Marie François Xavier Bichat (1771-1802), a pupil of the famous surgeon Pierre Joseph Desault (1744-1795). Bichat believed that surgery could provide a path to exact knowledge in medicine and physiology. According to Mark Altschule, such an emphasis on the surgical method had delayed the progress of French physiological research (Altschule 1984). So may have also the powerful influence of the patrons, or laboratory chiefs, who mainly constituted the membership of the Académie des Sciences and who controlled the research activities and even much of the thinking of their pupils and subordinates.

Many of these French scientists were engaged in endless philosophical debates, aligning themselves with fiercely held, but poorly defined beliefs about distinctions between the animate and inanimate world, convictions about the soul, the relationship of psychology to the laws of science and about purposefulness in organic structure. A rapidly dwindling number gathered under the banner of vitalism with the belief that life forms could not be understood in physical and chemical terms without involving an unknown "vital principle." Others, including

Bichat, veered toward vitalistic materialism, retaining a belief in the soul, but not involving it in thinking about physiology. Strict materialism, which denied man's spiritual character, was more common among the German physiologists. It had strong political implications in the revolutionary atmosphere of the mid-nineteenth century since it denied the divine right of kings.

The time was one of contention and confusion but it was also an intellectually fecund period (Temkin 1946). François Magendie (1783–1855), whose research made broad use of chemistry and pharmacology, established experimental physiology in France as an independent discipline, at the same time considering it to be fundamental to medical practice. His style of inquiry, inspired by the work of Albrecht von Haller (1708–1777) in Switzerland, according to John E. Lesch, was based largely on animal experimentation that yielded qualitative chemical data (Lesch 1977). Its character, more descriptive than quantitative, contrasted with the more "measuring" approach of the Germans who relied heavily on physics and technology.

During the early years of the nineteenth-century, Magendie taught as an *agrégé* in the Faculté de Médecine in Paris. He soon, however, became impatient with the dogmatism of medical practitioners and of medical school professors as well. He was troubled especially by the widely accepted isolation of clinical medicine from what he termed the "exact sciences" of physics and chemistry. Therefore, in 1813, he gave up his teaching post at the Faculté de Médecine in order to enter private practice and pursue his interest in studying the action of drugs. In 1821 the Académie des Sciences, having recognized physiology as a science, admitted Magendie as a physiologist, and soon established a prize in physiology. In 1830 Magendie was appointed director of a women's ward at Hôtel Dieu. Here he was able to conduct careful clinical trials in the evaluation of drugs, although most of his studies with natural alkaloids were performed on dogs.

Magendie's most famous pupil was Claude Bernard, a medical school classmate of Charles Richet's father, Alfred, who later became Bernard's personal physician. In 1839 both Bernard and Alfred competed successfully in the Concours de l'Internat, the selection of interns for the Paris hospitals. Bernard was assigned to Magendie's hospital ward as an intern. Magendie, impressed with the young man, took him into his department at the Collège de France as a student helper. Bernard had started as a pharmacist's apprentice but, like Richet, had initially been drawn to a career in literature. Indeed, he had written and published a few plays before entering medical school. Although his intellectual spark had attracted Magendie, Bernard was not a brilliant student. In fact, he had passed the baccalaureate examination with great difficulty. He did, however, write an acceptable doctoral thesis on gastric juice, but in 1844 when he applied for a teaching post in the Faculté de Médecine as *agrégé*, Bernard failed the examination. He decided then to become a country doctor. Circumstances intervened, however, by way of his marriage in 1845 to Fanny Martin, the daughter of a physician from whom he received a sufficient dowry to enable him to continue his physiological research. Therefore, in 1847, he returned to Magendie's laboratory at the Collège de France. According to Marilisa Juri, Claude Bernard, "in virtual exile (from clinical medicine) at the Collège de France, like Magendie before him, fought for a close collaboration between physicians and physiologists with the conviction that the experimental laboratory was a source of clinical medicine" (Juri 1965). After Magendie's death in 1855, Bernard was appointed to his chair at the Collège de France. In 1850, the year of Charles Richet's birth, Bernard applied for membership in the Académie des Sciences but was rejected. Nevertheless, in 1854 Bernard, having been awarded a doctorate in zoology in 1853, was appointed professor of general physiology of the faculty of science at the Sorbonne. In that year he was finally elected to the Académie des Sciences.

Bernard admitted no qualitative difference between normal and pathological processes. To him, disease was merely a matter of exaggerated, weakened or abolished physiological functions, while health was characterized by a balance of the internal organs, the "milieu intérieur" (Bernard 1952).[3] Bernard's methods of inquiry were simple and direct though highly ingenious. According to his biographer, Grmek, "the decisive turning point (in a piece of Bernard's research) was almost always his extraordinary capacity for noting in the course of an experiment a fact that did not accord with the prevailing theory" (Grmek 1966), a tactic often put to good use by Richet as well and one that Dr. Conan Doyle assigned as a "trademark" to Sherlock Holmes. Through the quality of Bernard's research and his highly effective efforts at promotion, physiology was rapidly achieving the national status of chemistry and physics. Despite Bernard's deep influence on Richet's thinking,

Richet had not applied to work with him because he had so many other students.

Scientists in French Government

The influence of the Académie des Sciences, coupled with that of the University, created to a large degree what Harry Paul called "The rise of the science empire in France" as prominent scholars and scientists continued to fill posts in the administrative departments of the government as well as in the Sénat and the Chambre des Deputés. (Paul 1985).

During the last third of the nineteenth-century French biological science began to receive urgently needed financial support from the government through the political activities of four outstanding scientists, all of whom more or less directly influenced Richet; Marcellin Berthelot (1827-1907), Paul Bert (1833-1886), Adolph Wurtz (1817-1884), and Jean Baptiste Dumas (1800-1884). The latter had actively promoted the work of Louis Pasteur (1822-1895). These men and their scientific predecessors, who had also served in the government as ministers or as senators or prominent members of the Chambre des Députés, made possible the financial support and public acceptance of the serious work in medical science of such as Claude Bernard and Louis Pasteur. Marcellin Berthelot, minister of education and Paul Bert, a member of the Chambre des Députés, with their almost fanatical belief in the capacity of science to free the human mind from dogma and error and ultimately to provide a rational social system, clearly contributed to the shaping of Richet's thoughts and convictions (Fox & Weisz 1980).

In his later years, Bernard turned his attention to philosophy. In this he may have stimulated Richet's interest in the field (See chapter 5). Although Bernard was influenced to some extent by the positivist philosophy of Auguste Comte (1798-1858) he rejected its dogmatic tenets and those of vitalism and materialism as well.[4] J.M.D. Olmsted, in his first (1938) biography of Bernard quotes from one of his unpublished essays that was called simply "Livre" (Olmsted 1938): "When a scientist pursues an investigation, taking for his starting point any particular philosophic system, he loses himself in regions too far removed from reality, or else the system gives his mind a misleading assurance and inflexibility." Olmsted adds, "He was at all times very emphatic about his dislike for what he called 'systems.'"[5] He refused his patronage impartially to the contemporary advocates of mechanism, materialism, and positivism, who scarcely disguised their eagerness to have his authority on their side. The materialists grew peevish, and openly attacked him in their journal, La Pensée Nouvelle for his refusal to take sides. Richet defended Bernard's position in an exchange of letters with a leading mechanist, the anthropologist Charles Jean-Marie Letourneau (1831-1902). "Claude Bernard is right to have avoided theories that cannot be proved," wrote Richet, "it is facts and not theories that physiologists and naturalists should be seeking." Concurring with Bernard, Richet wrote, "Physiology is finally disengaged from vitalism, religious or philosophic spiritualism, but that is not to thrust itself toward materialism. That would be to veer from Scylla to Charybdis."

From Bernard and from the naturalists, Henri Milne-Edwards (1800-1901), Lacaze-Duthiers (1821-1901) Richet may have acquired his way of approach to physiology, not merely asking "how does it work?" but, looking for an interpretation, "what is it all about?"

Richet's views and his approach to physiology were also influenced by the writings of the British physician-scientist and philosopher John Locke (1632-1704) that supported the concept that the brain's cognitive, emotional and reasoning functions are actuated by and dependent upon sensory input, a view that may have been borrowed from the French philosopher-scientist, Pierre Gassendi (1592-1655)[6] (Robertson 1971). The idea was adopted by Etienne Bonnot de Condillac (1715-1780) who is credited with importing Locke's views into Eighteenth-century French thought. In his Traité des Sensations published in 1754 in Denis Diderot's (1713-1784) thirty-four volume Encyclopédie published between 1752 and 1780, Condillac discussed the propositions that human understanding derives from the senses through attention, memory, comparison, judgment, and reflection (Condillac 1752). He and Diderot made that proposition the basis of a philosophical system for which his colleague Destutt de Tracy (1754-1836) coined the term Ideology to designate the scientific study of ideas. Ideology became a very powerful force in postrevolutionary France. Tracy considered it to be central to all sciences. He developed it into a republican and materialist doctrine, thus restricting its significance, but at the same time forging thereby a powerful weapon against Napoleon and the church (Kennedy 1979). Pierre Jean George Cabanis[7] (1757-1808) in his "Rapports du Physique et du Morale de l'Homme," first published in 1802, pursued and somewhat enlarged the concept of ideology as follows: "physiology, the analysis of ideas (ide-alogy) and ethics are but three branches of a single science which may justly be called 'The Science of man'" (Cabanis 1981). Richet, continu-ing Cabanis' line of thought, visualized the brain functioning as a dynamic interactive regulatory mechanism that activates and modulates all aspects of behavior, cognitive, emotional, volitional and visceral. Thus, he believed that the mind, like the body, must be subject to the laws of science.[R273]

Medical Education and Practice

Cabanis, echoing a theme of an eighteenth-century predecessor, Paul Joseph Barthez (1734-1806), had in 1878 expressed dissatisfaction over the pace of progress in French physiology and medicine in an essay, "The Degree of Certainty in Medicine," not published until ten years later after the Revolution. Cabanis insisted that "the true instruction of young doctors is not received from books, but at the bedside." Napoleon's physician Baron Jean Nicolas Corvisart (1755-1821) adopted this view and impressed it on his pupils, René Laennec (1781-1826) and Pierre Charles Louis (1787-1872), whose meticulous study of patients with the newly developed percussion and auscultation attracted droves of young physicians from the United States, Scandinavia, Great Britain, Germany, Austria, Spain, and Switzerland (Ackerknecht 1967).

While students were taught at the bedside, there was very little exposure to the basic sciences. In fact they were called "accessory" sciences among the medical faculty. Thus, there was a wide gap between the practitioners of medicine and the medical scientists not only in France but throughout Europe. Finally in the 1860s, according to George Weisz, the traditional complacency of the medical schools in France was chal-lenged by a demand for more supervision of the bedside clinical experi-ence of the medical students and for more science in medical education as well. The government's system, however, made such adjustments difficult. The hospital physicians were permitted to teach the medical students on the wards but were not part of the Faculté de Médecine and hence were ineligible to become professors. Professors were selected from faculty associates—the *agrégés*, those graduates who had success-fully completed a series of competitive examinations. They were con-trolled by the Ministry of Public Instruction. The hospital doctors, although drawn from the same pool of medical graduates, were under the Ministry of Interior. Neither group was much engaged in clinical or scientific research until after the Franco-Prussian War.

Basic science research took place mainly at the Faculté des Sciences at the Sorbonne and in the laboratories of the Collège de France where there were no classes for medical students. It was here that Richet was to conduct his first investigations in physiology.

The Collège de France had been founded in 1530 by François I, in part to protect the advance of science and scholarship from the heavy-handed and restrictive domination of the universities by the church. University teachers were often persecuted or even executed for presumed heretical views. At the Collège de France the emphasis was on study and inquiry. Its motto is "*omnia docet*," let all things be taught. A professor's function was to learn and lecture on new things. As Claude Bernard put it, "He should have his eyes turned toward the unknown, toward the future" (Olmsted 1938). Paradoxically, but perhaps not surprising, in view of the political confusion and lack of commitment to science at the medical school, the most distinguished academic physicians in France, including Napoleon's two physicians Jean Noel Halle (1754–1822), and Baron Jean Nicolas Corvisart held chairs in medicine at the Collège de France rather than at the university. Corvisart resurrected and popularized Leopold Edler von Auenbrugg's (1722–1809) percussion of the chest as an important aid to diagnosis. Laennec, a founder of clinical pathology and the inventor of the stethoscope, and Magendie also held professorships at the Collège de France.[8]

A practical concern for Richet, as it had been for Magendie and Bernard, was the lack of communication in the Faculté de Médecine between clinical medicine and the basic (accessory) medical sciences. Indeed, those identified as basic scientists were not welcome among those whose work it was to heal the sick. The role awaiting Richet was to move a step further toward the goal of Magendie and Bernard: to meld physiology with clinical medicine. Richet, who believed that physiology and medicine were parts of the same discipline, emphasized the point in his teaching and took the unique step of collaborating with clinicians in research.[9] Illustrative of his ecumenical convictions, Richet became a member and later president of the Académie de Médecine, of the Société de Biologie and of the Académie des Sciences. As a physiologist he repeatedly devoted his efforts to clinical problems, including the treatment of widely prevalent diseases. His motto was "Laboremus," like that of Sir William Osler (1849-1919) who preferred the English word "work" (Osler 1943).[10]

Notes

1. Tocqueville held that checks and balances were required to reconcile equality with freedom. He fought unsuccessfully for two legislative chambers instead of one parliamentary body. With the judicial system, however, he and his supporters were able to achieve more, including lifetime appointment of judges.

2. The idea of academies was not new. The probable forerunner of learned academies, and universities as well, was the library of Alexandria founded in the Third century B.C. under the rule of Ptolomy I. Academies of the Holy Roman Empire became functioning units of government under Charlemagne in 782 A.D.

3. Richet's elaborate theory that: "Life is a perpetual autoregulation, in adaption to the changing influences of the environment" quite clearly evolved from Bernard's formulation.

4. Comte proposed positiveness as a conceptual means of unifying the sciences, mathematics, astronomy, physics, chemistry, biology, and social sciences (Comte coined the word sociology). In a sense it provided the rationale for the formation of the Société de Biologie in 1848. The Société was founded by Claude Bernard with the histologist Charles Robin (1821-1885) and the physician-pathologist Pierre François Olive Rayer (1783-1867) who became its first president (Holmes 1974).

5. As Temkin points out, "In spite of his insistence on determinism in science, Claude Bernard did not believe in a purely mechanistic explanation of life." In his *Leçons sur les phénomènes de la vie*, written shortly before he died, he said, "The vital force directs phenomena that it does not produce; physical agents produce phenomena that they do not direct" (Temkin 1946).

6. Gassendi held views of the nature of matter and of life that were generally opposed to those of Descartes and were more in line with the empirical approach of Francis Bacon (1561-1626). He also elaborated on the concept of Democritus that motion is inherent in all matter. Locke may have become interested in Gassendi through François Bernier (1620-1687) whom he met during his sojourn in Paris. Bernier, according to Kenneth Dewhurst, was a physician and an orientalist who abridged and popularized Gassendi's philosophy (Dewhurst 1963).

7. Cabanis, the son of a jurist and botanist, was born in Rognac in southern France. He graduated in medicine at Paris in 1783 and later became identified with Condillac and Destutt de Tracy as a member of the Salon of Mme. Helvetius, widow of the philosopher, Claude Adrien Helvetius (1715-1771). The group came to be known as ideologues. The members included such notables as Condillac, Diderot, Thomas Jefferson (1743-1825), Benjamin Franklin (1706-1790), and Marie Jean Antoine Nicolas Caritat, Marquis de Condorcet (1743-1794), whose sister-in-law Cabanis married.

8. Laennec, a Catholic and royalist was appointed initially in competition with Magendie. Although he had, by his discovery of auscultation provided new access to the internal organs of patients, he did not believe that disease could be fully understood simply by the organic pathology. He wasn't a member of the vitalists but he opposed the philosophy of "organism" promoted by Leon-Louis Rostan

(1791–1886) who held "that all diseases could be reduced to physical or chemical changes in the solids or liquids of the body (Duffin 1988).

9. Nevertheless, the division between medical scientists and clinical investigators persisted in France in the support of research. It was clearly evident in 1963–64 when I served in Paris as a consultant to the Office of International Research of the National Institutes of Health. Investigators who studied animals were funded by mechanisms separate from those that supported investigators whose subjects were human beings. Since then the situation has changed dramatically so that French clinicians and basic scientists now collaborate freely. Richet, in his inaugural lesson as professor, had urged that clinical teaching be based on and joined with studies in the basic sciences twenty-five years before a similar proposal was made in the United States by the influential Flexner report (Flexner 1912).

10. William Osler the first professor of medicine at Johns Hopkins University (1886) was famous worldwide for his diagnostic acumen and his bedside teaching methods. From 1912 when he left Hopkins and until his death he served as Regius Professor of Medicine at Oxford.

3

Education in Medicine and Science
1869–1878

After entering the University, Charles continued to live with his parents, but he resisted meeting many of the people his father wanted him to know, preferring his old comrades who enjoyed the opera, poetry, and literature but also parties, dances, and visits to the music halls. He continued to write plays, stories, and poetry, often in collaboration with his friend Paul Fournier under the pseudonym Charles Epheyre, a combination of initials F and R.

Medical School

The major event during Richet's years in medical school was the interruption caused by the Franco-Prussian War of 1870. It affected him deeply and reinforced the pacifistic teachings of his grandfather. Charles was first assigned as a guard at the Invalides and later to an ambulance corps at Versailles. He was appalled by the slaughter of young French soldiers and the accompanying low birth rate in France. Years later, in a speech before the Académie de Médecine he said, "La question de la natalité n'est pas pour les Français la question la plus importante, c'est la seule."[R566 1] Richet attributed the low birth rate in France to economic pressures, especially the high cost of raising children. He proposed that to reverse the trend the French government should provide generous cash subsidies to pregnant mothers and continue to help them financially through the childhood of their offspring.

After the war Charles completed his course of studies but his grades in medical school did not match his fine record at the Lycée. He continued living at his parents' home but studied little and spent much time partying with his friends. When his father caught him dropping notes on a string through the window to a chambermaid in the apartment below with whom young Charles had established an intimate relationship, he insisted that he move to an apartment closer to the medical school.

During his internship at the Salpêtrière in 1872 Richet's scholarly extracurricular interests were again in evidence. He began the first French translation from the Latin of William Harvey's (1578–1657) classical description of the circulation of the blood, *De Motu Cordis*, originally published in 1628.[R 41]

Hypnotism and the Occult

Richet's interest in Latin was soon supplemented by a powerful preoccupation with psychic phenomena, including hypnotism. His fascination with hypnotism began when at the age of sixteen he had observed an entertainer named Cannelle put a "very pretty woman" to sleep and showed her to be apparently unable to feel pain (Unp). Richet promptly tried hypnosis on a young friend of his sister in the course of a parlor game and thus satisfied himself of the authenticity of the phenomenon. He then tried unsuccessfully to persuade his friend and teacher Henri Liouville to let him hypnotize patients at Hôtel Dieu, his father's hospital. He later had the opportunity to practice hypnosis during his clinical rotation on the wards of the Salpêtrière that were under the direction of the famous neurologist, Jean Louis Martin Charcot (1825–1893). Richet encountered a patient, a sixteen-year-old girl with an hysterical contracture of one arm. He successfully hypnotized her so that her disability disappeared, but it soon recurred. Repeatedly he was able to eliminate her contracture with hypnosis, and repeatedly it recurred soon afterward.

The following year (1873) Richet successfully competed for an appointment as "*interne des hopitaux de Paris*," roughly equivalent to a residency in the United States. He began his work with the surgeon, Leon Clément Lefort (1829–1893), who was in charge of a female ward at Hôpital Beaujon. Having little interest in the routine surgical problems, Richet began treating the neurotic patients with hypnosis, which he called "*somnambulisme provoqué*." "My experiences with hypnotism," he wrote, "determined my career. No longer uncertain between medicine and surgery, having tasted experimentation, I realized it was my path and I decided early in 1873 to become a psychophysiologist" (Unp).

In 1875, against the advice of his father, who said that such a focus of interest would ruin his reputation, or nip it before it budded, Richet published an article *Le Somnambulisme Provoqué*[R2] (i.e. hypnosis).[2] that preceded by three years the first publication of Charcot on the use of hypnosis in hysterical patients (Charcot 1878). In the meantime Richet's findings were acknowledged and confirmed by the famous physiologist Rudolf Peter Heinrich Heidenhain (1834-1897) in Germany whose major discoveries related to the mechanisms of glandular secretion and kidney function but who also wrote a book on animal magnetism published in 1880 (Heidenhain 1880). On page 58 of the English translation he refers to correspondence with Richet and cites Richet's 1875 publication. Thus Richet's work and his priority were recognized prior to his completing his medical studies.[3]

In 1886 Hippolyte Bernheim (1840-1919), a professor at the Faculté de Médecine in Nancy and a professional rival of Charcot, published a book on the uses of hypnotism in medical therapy. In it he credited Richet's 1875 publication with not only having preceded Charcot's work, but with having called attention for the first time to the therapeutic potential of hypnosis (Bernheim 1889). Bernheim, following the idea of the Scottish surgeon and hypnotist James Braid (1795-1860), who had concluded that hypnosis consists of suggestion, not sleep, was able to reproduce in patients many of the phenomena of hypnosis by simple suggestion. Still prior to the publications of Charcot on the subject, another young doctor named Ruault had picked up Richet's interest in hypnosis at the Salpêtrière. Richet wrote that he was "in reality the one who, with his beautiful experiments, showed Charcot what somnambulism is. Charcot published the work without even mentioning Ruault . . . I had the same experience"[4] (Unp).

Another who acknowledged Richet's priority in the medical uses of hypnotism was Wilhelm Max Wundt (1832-1920) a student of William James (1842-1910) and one of the earliest academic psychologists. Wundt established the world's first laboratory of experimental psychology in Leipzig. He cited Richet's work on hypnotism in his book, *Hypnotism and Suggestion* (Wundt 1893). While he praised Richet and acknowledged the validity of hypnotism and its possible usefulness in therapy, he considered it unsuitable for experimental research because of its inconsistency.

While still serving his residency with Lefort, Richet, having acquired an interest in clairvoyance as well as hypnotism published an article in a lay journal the *Revue Philosophique*, "La Suggestion Mentale et le Calcul des Probabilités" in which he tested the statistical validity of clairvoyance. [R15] Using the laws of probability, he calculated the likelihood that extrasensory perception actually exists, as claimed when a person correctly identifies playing cards turned over by another person in secret. He concluded that repeatedly successful identification of the cards could not be a matter of chance. Richet's priority in this regard was acknowledged in Mauskopf and McVaugh's 1979 review of Joseph Banks Rhine's (1895-1980) work on extrasensory perception (Mauskopf and McVaugh 1980).

With reference to Richet's convictions concerning clairvoyance, Wundt wrote that, "although Richet's findings merited attention because of his solid work in physiology, they force us to conclude that there is a world of natural laws and another world of spirits that defy and disrupt those laws." Furthermore, he averred that what mediums have successfully predicted are not major events but minor happenings in someone's family or in the identification of playing cards from a distance. He wondered how such relatively trivial matters could have so occupied the efforts of a man [Richet] "otherwise full of wisdom" (Wundt 1893).

Opting for a Career in Science

During his course in chemistry in the laboratory of Charles Adolph Wurtz, Richet and his friend Henri Hermite, the nephew of the famous mathematician,[6] happened to see a posted announcement of forthcoming qualifying examinations to work toward a science degree as well as the MD. As Richet recalled in his *Souvenirs d'un Physiologiste*, "I was too naive, too ignorant and perhaps too lazy to profit from my opportunities (in Wurtz's laboratory), but more valuable than the experiments were the contacts with distinguished people who visited."[R736] Richet and Hermite decided to apply. Although in Richet's day very few medical students sought also to work toward the science degree, applicants were, nevertheless, required to compete so that at least one person could be rejected. At first only Richet and Hermite were applying but fortunately a third applicant appeared, a Romanian named Angelescu whom both of them defeated.

Richet's next step was to select a field of study. Recalling his enjoyment of the zoology courses in the Faculté des Sciences taught by Lacaze Duthiers and Milne Edwards he chose to work on the comparative physiology of muscular contraction in invertebrates. He now needed to find a suitable laboratory in which to work. Auguste Béclard (1817–1887), the perpetual secretary of the Académie de Médecine, professor of physiology and dean of the Faculté de Médecine, had very little time to spend in the two small rooms that constituted his laboratory. Richet therefore chose to work in the laboratory of Marey[7] at the Collège de France. As noted in chapter 1, Marey was particularly well known for his development of graphic methods, originally introduced by Carl Ludwig in Leipzig with whom Marey had studied.

Although Richet was eager for instruction and experience in graphic methods and later was able to apply them to great advantage in physiological studies, he was not handy or skillful with them at first so Marey, a man almost obsessed with his graphics, paid little attention to him. Richet, therefore, began his muscle project pretty much on his own, beginning with the musculature of the tail and pincers of the crayfish.

Richet's study of the crayfish was interrupted for a time when the surgeon, Aristide Auguste Stanislas Verneuil (1823–1895), a former assistant to Richet's father, presented him an unusual opportunity to study the function of the stomach in man.

Gastric Juice and Gastric Sensation

Having been called to see a fifteen-year-old boy known as Marcellin, who had acquired an esophageal stricture from accidentally having swallowed potassium hydroxide, Verneuil was encouraged to perform a gastrostomy to bypass his patient's occluded esophagus. A successful surgical gastrostomy on a patient with an obstructive carcinoma of the esophagus had been reported the previous year by a British surgeon named Jones (Jones 1875). Verneuil accomplished the operation on Marcellin in 1876, leaving him with a gastric fistula, an opening through the skin of his abdomen directly into the stomach (Verneuil 1876).

Responsive to young Richet's ambition toward research, and perhaps sensitive to the opportunity to gain the older Richet's favor, Verneuil sent a message to Charles, who at the time was on vacation in the Middle East. He had reached Egypt when he received Verneuil's message, "Come immediately. Since you are interested in physiology you will have a magnificent example of gastric physiology to study."

Richet welcomed the opportunity and quickly returned to Paris. He had already begun a thesis for his medical degree on experimental and clinical studies of sensation. He therefore began his study of Marcellin by addressing himself to gastric sensibility and included his observations in his thesis.[R 6] Richet ascertained that Marcellin could not appreciate touch in his stomach, that cold fluids elicited pain and that alcohol caused a sensation of heat. Marcellin could not tell whether his stomach was full or empty. Very rapid filling or emptying of the stomach, however, was consistently associated with hiccough.[R 6]

Richet's thesis for the M.D. degree on sensation became his first published physiological inquiry. Thereafter he maintained a continuing interest in sensation and other properties of the nervous system. Some of the experiments relating to pain that were reported in his thesis were included in a book *La Douleur*[R 9] and in papers that appeared in *Revue Scientifique*,[R 402] and *Dictionnaire de Physiologie*.[R 418] He described hyperalgesia associated with inflammation and noted that the extent of the spread of referred pain was related to its intensity. He also marshalled evidence for a center in the brain for pain "probably located near the internal capsule" and reported on the actions of analgesic drugs. He noted that some of them provided relief by inhibiting the transmission of pain impulses, that others impaired memory of the pain and still others induced a feeling of detachment and indifference to pain. He also documented the significance of experience, culture and psychological state in determining the intensity of pain perceived[8] following a uniform stimulus, as well as the emotional and behavioral responses to it. In these texts he clearly indicated, as he had during his internship with Lefort, his commitment to psychophysiology as a career choice.

Returning to his work on the stomach and recognizing the need to do chemical analyses on the gastric juice of Marcellin, Richet obtained access to the laboratory of Professor Berthelot, located near that of Marey at the Collège de France. Berthelot was a widely renowned chemist who could provide the necessary tools and advice for Richet's work.

Verneuil's patient, Marcellin, came daily to Richet's borrowed laboratory. Direct access to the stomach of a young man who was healthy except for his benign stricture enabled Richet to make a unique contribution. There had been no previously published physiological studies of patients with surgically produced gastric fistulae.[9] After demonstrating that his subject's esophageal obstruction was complete, Richet went on to study gastric juice obtained from the patient's stomach without contamination by saliva. His analysis of the gastric juice became the central topic of his thesis for the Ph.D. degree (Docteur ès science).[R 13,14]

While studying his fistulous subject, Marcellin, Richet had actually observed the "psychic phase" of gastric secretion, the acceleration of gastric acid secretion with appetite and tasting, prior to its discovery by Ivan Petrovitch Pavlov (1849–1936). He had reported that gastric acidity increased after he gave the boy some candies to chew which, of course, could not traverse the occluded esophagus to reach the stomach. But he failed to appreciate the significance of his observation. Later, in *Souvenirs d'un Physiologiste*, Richet told of his lapse of perceptiveness: "too often" he wrote, "we can only see what we are looking for; absurd in the extreme because one must observe whatever happens, even what one does not expect, *especially* what one does not expect."[R 736]

The studies of Marcellin thoroughly confirmed Beaumont's finding that hydrochloric acid is the principal acid in the gastric juice, originally identified in the secretion of human stomachs by William Prout (1785–1850) (Prout 1824). Richet was the first to show that to some extent HCl was linked to nitrogen-containing organic substances. Thus, the stomach contains both "free" and "combined acid."[R 17,18] He also discovered that the acidity of the gastric juice increased during the process of gastric digestion and further observed that the concentration of HCl was greater in carnivores than in the herbivores.[R 37] When Richet presented his findings to the Société de Biologie, he provoked the "enormous indignation" of Jean Baptiste Vincent Laborde (1831–1903) a politically powerful physician and physiologist, a member of the Faculté de Médecine. Laborde had published a paper contradicting the conclusions of Prout and Beaumont that HCl is present in the gastric juice. Richet reported that in challenging his methods, Laborde "declared in violent language that I had fallen into error" (Unp).

Further Studies of Gastric Acidity at a Marine Laboratory

One day when Richet encountered Claude Bernard in the courtyard of the Collège de France, Bernard, whose thesis for the MD degree had dealt with the gastric juice, and who had created gastric fistulae in animals to study digestion, advised Richet to pursue further his studies in fishes because of the high acidity of their gastric secretions (Bernard 1839). Bernard's suggestion led Richet to the seashore at Le Havre where he undertook the study of the gastric juice of sharks with the help of Gustave Lennier.[R 56] Lennier, who had made important studies of the Seine estuary, was curator of a natural history museum that occupied a building that had been a museum of art.

Marine laboratories had begun to be recognized as useful for research in comparative physiology.[10] Paul Bert made a visit to the Le Havre and directed one of his assistants, Dr. Paul Régnard, a classmate of Richet, to construct a laboratory of marine biology above an aquarium on St. Roche square. Lennier, who had installed the aquarium in 1869, and Dr. Gilbert, a local physician, helped Régnard establish the institution where, not only Bert and Richet, but Louis Olivier, Paul Loye, Jean Paul Langlois and many other physiologists came to work. So had Prince Albert I of Monaco (1848–1922) a distinguished marine biologist in his own right.[11] Prince Albert provided much of the funding for what became l'Institut Oceanographique with Régnard as director. At Le Havre in about 1881 Richet met Jean Paul Langlois (1862–1923) who was serving a medical residency at the local hospitals. Langlois soon joined Richet in Paris as his laboratory chief and became his collaborator in research throughout Richet's remaining years.

Richet came frequently to Le Havre to pursue his studies of the gastric juice of marine animals. To test its acidity he used phenolphthalein, a colored indicator of acidity recently developed in Germany by fellow student in Berthelot's laboratory, Gustave Bouchard (1842–1918). Richet also used phenolphthalein in his studies of the fermentation of milk.[R 18] He first added gastric juice to the milk and later studied the effects of myriad substances and conditions on the process of lactic fermentation, a phenomenon that continued to engage his attention off and on for the next fifty years.

Now, however, his task was to complete his thesis for the science degree based on his studies of gastric juice in Berthelot's laboratory. That done, he sat for his examination for the degree, *Docteur ès Sciences*. Claude Bernard had recently died and his place at the Sorbonne had been taken by Paul Bert. Bert, Edmond Hébert (1812–1890) and Milne-Edwards, dean of the Faculté des Sciences, were the examiners. Richet was awarded the degree despite his failure to answer a question posed by Bert concerning the geology of La Hève, near Le Havre where Richet had made his studies of the gastric juice of fish.

Richet earned his degree in the basic medical sciences just before physiology had made its escape from the domination of anatomy, as discussed in chapter 2. A new association with chemistry had evolved. Both Magendie and Bernard had relied heavily on chemistry in their work. Richet's early experience in Berthelot's laboratory had left an especially deep impression on him. He recalled Berthelot as a cold and distant person but one who was interested in his pupils and generous with his time. Richet concluded his work in Berthelot's laboratory with a high regard for the man and deep conviction of the importance of chemistry to physiology. Richet also venerated the great chemist, Lavoisier and was to work a few years later on the topic of Lavoisier's great contribution, the relationship of respiration to internal combustion.

Muscles and Nerves

Before having completed his studies of the chemistry of the gastric juice, Richet had resumed work of the crayfish muscles in the laboratory of Marey. He demonstrated that nerves and muscles responded to excitation in much the same fashion whether the stimulus be electrical, chemical, or mechanical but he noted a difference in the pattern of muscular contraction of the tail and pincer of the crayfish.[R 43] The movements of the tail were rapid and not sustained, while the pincers contracted more slowly and maintained a firm grip over long periods. Moreover, he observed that the fast muscles of the tail were white and less capable of sustained contraction than the reddish more vascular muscles of the pincers. This was an important contribution to muscle physiology. Later workers discovered that fast, poorly vascular muscle fibers derive short term energy from the breakdown of glycogen, while the slow fibers that are highly vascular, and hence red, derive more sustained energy from oxidative metabolism of glucose. With his taste for the spectacular, and having recently read an 1859 article in Latin in *Pflügers Archiv* by M. Hermann on muscular contraction, (Hermann 1859) Richet published in Latin a short report of his work on the crayfish muscles in *Pflügers Archiv*.[R 114] Of that achievement he wrote in his *Mémoires*, "I think mine was the only published work in Latin by a living physiologist." In it he referred to earlier work by Luchsinger who, on electrically stimulating the muscles of the crayfish claw, found that "a feeble excitation causes dilatation, while a strong one causes constriction" (Luchsinger 1882). In a later publication Richet cited Hermann's work.[R7]

Working with the same animal preparation, Richet further discovered the phenomenon of summation, the effectiveness of a series of weak stimuli that individually are insufficient to achieve firing of a nerve or contraction of a muscle. Richet also observed summation of sensory stimuli in the skin. That is, a stimulus of insufficient strength to be felt when applied singly would elicit pain if it were delivered repeatedly in a rapid volley. His next objective was to ascertain whether or not other sensations would respond to summation. Choosing to work first on vision, he required a specially calibrated instrument with which to vary intensity and duration of exposure to a beam of light. He approached a young electrical engineering student, Antoine Breguet (1851-1882) a friend of his cousin, Robert Girard, to collaborate on the project. Antoine, a member of a family of famous watchmakers had recently discontinued his studies at L'Ecole Polytechnique to run his father's business. Breguet fabricated the required instrument and, with Richet, demonstrated that an intensity of light, not visible during a brief exposure, became visible if the exposure were prolonged.[R45]

By 1878 Richet had begun to work in the laboratory of Edme-Felix-Alfred Vulpian (1826-1887), a famous experimental pathologist and physiologist whose activities were centered chiefly on the nervous system. Vulpian a long time pupil of Charcot had become chief of a service at the Salpêtrière. Richet extended to the brain his earlier investigations on summation of electrical impulses applied to both motor and sensory nerves. In crayfish and frogs he demonstrated that a single electrical stimulus, insufficient to provoke a muscular response when applied to the brain, produced vigorous movement of an extremity when administered to the brain repetitively at the rate of forty impulses per second.[R81] Thus, he demonstrated that summation occurred in neurons of the brain as well as in the periphery. For his thesis to qualify for a faculty post Richet chose the anatomy and physiology of the surface structures (convolutions) of the brain of animals and man. He dedicated the thesis, "Structure des Convolutions Cérébrales" to the neuroscientist and anthropologist Pierre Paul Broca (1824-1880), who identified a site in the brain required for speech, and J.M. Charcot.[R16]

Several years later with Broca's son, André (1863-1925), another student of Vulpian, Richet applied stimulating electrodes directly to the cortex of the dog's brain in the region of the Rolandic convolution, the site where the nerve cells of the brain initiate movements of the extremities. This work led them to the discovery of a refractory period (an interval of unresponsiveness to a new stimulus delivered shortly after a response) in the brain similar to that which Marey had discovered for the heart.

Richet continued his collaboration with André Broca and in 1897 they reported experiments in which they were able to manipulate the length of the refractory period in nerve cells of the brain by changing the ambient temperature and by anesthesia with chloralose. They showed that the refractory period was governed by the time required to "restore electrical equilibrium," the repolarization of the nerve cell. Marey arranged for the work to be presented before the Académie des Sciences.[R 407]

Having now completed the requirements for a teaching post, Richet presented himself for appointment as *agrégé*, or faculty associate in the basic sciences. He was to have had two competitors, Charles Albert François Franck (1849-1921) and Charles Rémy. Franck withdrew, having written to Richet that it would be futile to present himself against the son of one of the professors. Richet eliminated Rémy by showing that his thesis on pituitary secretions contained illustrations plagiarized from an existing publication. The reduced competition was fortunate for Richet, since he had again done poorly in his oral examination. Following it, Marie Philibert Sappey (1810-1896) the professor of anatomy, said to him, "here you are an associate in anatomy, but you know nothing about it. Promise me that you will learn because you will have examinations to pass later on." Richet promised in good faith to study anatomy, but he spared little time from his many other interests to do so.

After successfully completing his examination for the science degree in 1877 Richet traveled to the Château de Stors to visit his grandfather Renouard.[12]

His fiancee, Amélie Aubry,[13] had dreamt that Richet's mother and Renouard were at the château and that Renouard was sick. On his arrival there Richet found that Renouard had died suddenly after an intense chest pain. "This was a terrible blow for all of us" wrote Richet, "but for me, perhaps, more than others. I have already said that my grandfather was an inspiration of my life. I was proud of him and I felt his great spirit close to me. His counsel, his lessons and his example were always important to me. Often I asked myself what the ideal of perfection is. It is my grandfather Charles Renouard" (Unp).

The death of his beloved grandfather seemed to awaken in Charles Richet a greater sense of purpose than had been evident before. He applied himself more seriously to his work. According to Gabriel, however, there had been some change in his grandfather, Charles Richet, a bit earlier when his vacation in Egypt was interrupted by the letter from Verneuil giving him the opportunity to study Marcellin. At that time he seems to have become imbued with ambition for academic distinction and a desire to become a savant.

Notes

1. The birth rate is not the main concern for the French; it is the only concern.
2. Since hypnosis was generally considered to be a form of sleep, the term was used synonymously with somnambulism.
3. Charcot's interest in hysteria and his use of hypnosis in its treatment intrigued young Sigmund Freud (1856-1939) who was just starting a practice in Vienna. A travel grant from his university enabled him to study with Charcot at the Salpêtrière from October 1885 - February 1886. He later translated several of Charcot's publications into German. It was the effects of hypnosis in hysterical patients that led Freud to his concept of the unconscious and of repression of emotional conflicts as a cause of neurosis (Charcot 1878; Richer & Charcot 1883).
4. Richet felt that he had been denied credit for several of his discoveries, but especially for being the first to induce passive immunity discussed in chapter 5.
5. His method was to estimate the probability of each of a series of successful tries and then multiply the probabilities together to get an overall probability. Discussed by Mauskopf and McVaugh, the technique hardly matches the rigor of modern statistics (Mauskopf & McVaugh 1980). Richet's interest in clairvoyance and other presumed psychical abilities was consonant with his view that all mental functions, as part of psychology, are explainable by natural laws and are hence potentially a part of physiology.
6. Charles Hermite (1822-1902) professor of Higher Algebra at the Sorbonne, after whom the Law of Reciprocity was named, was credited with being the first to solve fifth degree equations.
7. After Claude Bernard's death Marey was elected to his place in the Académie des Sciences in 1878. Paul Bert and Charcot were his two unsuccessful competitors.
8. These observations provide an early example of Richet's remarkable sensitivity to clues and his ability to recognize their significance. A clear distinction between perception and reaction to pain was not formulated until the work of Wolff, Hardy & Goodell sixty years later (Wolff 1940,1941).
9. There had, however, been several important studies of humans with accidentally acquired gastric fistulae. Richet was aware of the work of William Beaumont (1785-1853) on Alexis St. Martin, published in 1833 (Beaumont 1833). In 1530 Matthew Cornax, a Viennese professor of medicine and physician to the Holy

Roman Emperor, Ferdinand I, had reported the case of a man who, while hunting, was wounded in the abdomen by a stake (Cornax 1564). It penetrated his stomach and produced a permanent gastric fistula. A Viennese physician, Jacob Helm (1761–1831) reported observations on a woman with a gastric fistula acquired as a consequence of the bursting of an abscess of her abdominal wall (Helm 1801). Napoleon's physician, Baron Jean Nicolas Corvisart des Marets with the collaboration of Leroux, published a study of the chemical composition of gastric juice obtained from a forty-seven-year-old woman who, like the patient of Cornax, and acquired a traumatic fistula (Corvisart & Leroux 1802). In carefully documenting the extent to which a great variety of foods underwent gastric digestion, Beaumont contributed to the still embryonic science of nutrition. He also made the first experimental observation on the effects of emotionally stressful experiences on the stomach (Beaumont 1833). Finally, he provided the first systematic description of the muscular movements of the gastric wall. Beaumont's greatest contribution, however, was his exemplary method of investigating his human subject and of recording his data.

10. The first European marine laboratory was founded in 1843 in Ostend, Belgium by Pierre Joseph Van Beneden (1809–1894) Professor of Natural Science at Louvain. The oldest of the French marine laboratories was founded by Jacques Marie Cyprien Victor Coste (1807–1873) at Concarneau in Finistère on the southern coast of Brittany in the mid 1850s. By far the most famous, however, was the one established by the German, Anton Felix Dohrn (1840–1909) in Naples in 1872. It was directed thereafter by three generations of Dohrns, Anton, his son and grandson, all of whom retained their German citizenship.

11. Prince Albert had established one of the world's earliest marine biology research laboratories in Monte Carlo. He also hosted biology trips on his yacht, the Princesse Alice, in which he had installed a research laboratory and holding tanks for collected specimens.

12. Stors was a village in the Commune of L'Isle-Adam on the river Oise. The château was built in the seventeenth-century by the Marquis de Verderonne and was later bought by the last Prince of Conti in 1786. He, in turn, sold it to the brother of Louis XVI who later became Louis XVIII. The château was confiscated during the revolution and was eventually bought by a descendent of the duc de Valmy who was soon bankrupt from gambling. In 1860 he sold the château to a financier named Casimir Chevreux, husband of Richet's aunt Hortense Girard. Their daughter Louise married Mr. Guillemin. The Guillemins' daughter Madeleine, in 1873, married the grandson of Maréchal Lannes, Count Gustave de Montebello, who became French ambassador to Russia. Madeleine ultimately inherited Stors which still belongs to the Montebello family. I am indebted to Mme. Montebello de Baecque, the great granddaughter of Madeleine and the Count, for this information and for a photograph of the château.

13. Richet's engagement and marriage to Amélie are described in the next chapter.

4

The Competitive Young Physiologist
1878–1887

Once he became a member of the faculty Richet lost no time in assuming the role of savant, or scientist-scholar. In his book *Le Savant*, published in 1923 as part of a series of essays by leaders in politics, religion and other fields of activity in France,[R 649] Richet described what he considered to be a code of proper attitudes and behavior for a savant. He found the qualities especially well exemplified in Claude Bernard and Louis Pasteur, about whom he wrote, "they were as audacious in hypothesis as they were rigorous in experiment . . . but happily they had something else which gave impulse to their genius and made their work fruitful. They had enthusiasm." Richet contended that with virtues such as these, "the happiness and the future of humanity will depend upon science."

Charles Richet was certainly audacious and he had enthusiasm in full measure, but he was, perhaps, less disciplined, less sharply focused on each of the areas of his investigation than were his two idols. As his grandson, Gabriel expressed it, "He painted with a broad brush and had little interest in figures. He investigated whatever seemed intriguing to him and to some extent one study suggested another. His style was to initiate an enquiry, often with an imaginative strategy, and pursue it far enough to satisfy his curiosity but not as far as it could lead him. In this respect he was intellectually restless and, in a sense, Olympian as he left the gaps for others to fill." Nevertheless, a careful look at the total production of Richet's laboratory work will reveal a common theme, concern with the biological significance of an observation or discovery, often at the expense of wrapping up loose ends. It appears to have been his surprising versatility and his capacity for synthesis that contributed most to Richet's self esteem.

According to his sons, Charles and Alfred, and his two grandsons, Gabriel and Denis, much of Richet's satisfaction came from being the center of attention. He especially enjoyed astounding people with his brilliance and breadth of knowledge. His erudition and his accomplishments aroused admiration and deference among his colleagues, but rarely affection. While he deeply admired many of his senior colleagues and teachers, even venerated some of them, Richet seemed somehow to remain emotionally detached. He explained his lack of close involvement with the distinguished savants in whose laboratories he had worked and for whom he had affection and admiration: "perhaps because I was independent in character and in circumstance I was never really the pupil—the intimate disciple of anyone. I worked in the laboratories of Wurtz, Berthelot, Marey and, Vulpian. It is my regret that I never was their collaborator . . . of my own obscure and youthful work they knew practically nothing."

Richet's tendency toward aloofness was evident in his deportment among his colleagues on the faculty. His behavior was meticulously correct but he did not seek close relationships with many of them. His model savant seems to have been his friend and Nobel prize-winning physicist, Gabriel Lippmann (1845-1921) whom he characterized as follows, "He was a man of admirable serenity and scrupulous conscience. At once a worker and a dreamer, he followed a lonely path with lofty thoughts. With modesty he fled from honors and other banalities of daily life, seeking instead the esthetically pleasing and the best products of the spirit. Although kindly and attentive to others, he nevertheless listened with one ear, being unwilling to abandon his own thoughts for those of the speaker"—"a very legitimate attitude," added Richet.[R649]

In choosing companions outside the faculty Richet sought characteristics somewhat at variance with the ones he admired in a savant. Those whom he accepted as friends had the qualities of independence, humor and aesthetic appreciation that he found in Antoine Breguet with whom he worked on the phenomenon of summation of visual stimuli and whom he described as follows: "From the moment we met, as with Emanuel (Bourdon) and Robert Girard, I was entranced, overcome, charmed; from the beginning we understood each other. Tall, slender, distinguished with a charming face, a sympathetic voice and irrepressible gaiety, he exerted on all who saw him an irresistible attraction. Without wishing to denigrate my friends I must say that Antoine Breguet was one of the most remarkable characters I have known. He did what he wished, played comedy and recited verses in a delicious manner. His memory was perfect and in mathematics and physics he had an ingeniousness that always astonished me" (Unp).

Richet had very little time for people who were neither charming nor witty, nor polished, nor intellectual, nor loyal to friends, nor devoted to France. He was convinced of the superiority of Western Europeans in general and of Frenchmen in particular. In keeping with what he gathered from Darwin's writings, Richet concluded that it was natural for the British to rule in India simply because of their intellectual superiority. He added that he had nothing against Indians, that he was merely stating a scientific fact.

Grandson Gabriel recalled an incident at Carqueiranne when, during a tactical exercise, a Senegalese company was billeted there: "The officers, some of whom were black, lodged for the night in the château. When it was time for dinner, however, [Richet] concocted another commitment so he would not have to sit at table with them." His hauteur often extended to his adversaries and sometimes to his colleagues.

Marriage

Richet's recreational social life was spent mainly in the company of the men who had been friends from his childhood but he loved the company of beautiful women, especially the high born. Although highly attractive to women, Richet, previous to his marriage, seems to have had no serious or lasting romantic attachments. As he put it, "I had had neither desire nor distaste for marriage, but I had taken no steps toward it; neither had my parents." The issue was raised thanks to a chain of events that began with Richet's father, Alfred, having operated upon a wealthy businessman named Maurice Aubry. Charles was given the task of sitting with Aubry during the postoperative period to make sure everything was going well. Much of the time was spent in what Richet considered an interesting but somewhat disputatious dialogue about politics, Aubry being a royalist and Richet, of course, a republican. After Aubry's recovery his wife, Adèle, invited the Richet family for dinner at their luxurious apartment. She had included a young woman named Thérèse Donon whom she thought would make a good wife for Charles. He came bringing flowers, arrived a little too early, and sat with the men who were waiting in the smoking room. After dinner, as was customary, Charles had to submit to a sort of inquisition by the girls' mother, Madame Donon. She had great difficulty in understanding how he could devote his efforts both to literature and to science. He explained that he was an independent soul: "I emphasized to her that I always do what I please and I would never commit myself to something. I write in verse when I wish or in prose. I could see that I was compromising my chances for marriage but that didn't matter" (Unp). Madame Donon, of course, did not give her consent to an engagement.

At this point, Felix Aubry, whose wife had died some years before reminded his sister-in-law, Adèle that his own daughter, Amélie, might be an appropriate wife for Richet. Again there were the same sort of interviews, one with Mademoiselle Duhamel whom Felix had hired as a tutor for Amélie after the death of his wife. Richet described Mademoiselle Duhamel as "quite frightening, very strict and meticulous. It was necessary for me to explain to her my political and religious opinions, which inspired in me a considerable fear. It was not only her of whom I was afraid but also my future brother-in-law Albert Aubry and my fiancee herself" (Unp). The religious problem began to stand in the way because Albert was strictly religious and deeply devoted to the Jesuits and so was Mademoiselle Duhamel. Even Amélie felt the need to discuss with Charles the matter of religion. Again Richet went through pretty much the same explanation he had made to Madame Donon, but emphasized that, although he had no belief at all in the teachings of the church, and hence had no religion, he nevertheless respected the religion of others and would not interfere at all with his wife pursuing her religion or the religious education of the children. The terms were accepted and the marriage took place on the 27th of August 1878 at the Church of Saint Eustache on rue Ste. Cécile near the Aubry's home at 35 rue du Faubourg Poissonnière.

The Aubry family had come originally from Mirecourt, a little town in the Vosges, well known worldwide for "lutherie," the manufacture of stringed instruments. Amélie's father, Felix was born in 1812. His father owned a small bank and his mother operated a small lace business in Nancy. As a youth Felix traveled around the area in a horse drawn wagon selling his mother's lace. He later came to Paris where he worked for a shopkeeper named Peigné and married his daughter, Amélie's mother. He soon created his own bank. Through his banking activities and his other enterprises, Aubry contributed substantially to the development of the French economy. Amélie was their second child. Her older brother, a graduate of the Ecole Polytechnique, was killed in the Franco-Prussian War near Vendôme. After Amélie, the Aubrys had two more children. One, Adèle, died of puerperal infection; the other, Albert became a successful businessman.

Because he generally opposed the clergy and the dogmas of the church, Richet found it difficult to adjust to the deep religious beliefs of his wife, Amélie. He stood by his promise to Mme. Donon, however, and, as he wrote in his *Mémoires*

> I think that I never interfered with my wife's devout practice of her religion. When I say never, there was an exception, a moment of anger very early in our marriage about which I have great regret because I was completely wrong. When we were taking our honeymoon we were in Rome and my wife, without consulting me, requested an audience with the Pope. I think it was Pope Pius IX, but to appear before the Pope a certain costume was required, a mantle over the head, and when I saw her disguised in this fashion to receive the benediction from the Pope, I was suddenly seized by a fit of anger and I remember that I threw a book that I was holding violently on the floor. It was absurd, and after I had a chance to reflect, I found that this was stupid. After all, one is responsible only for one's self. I think that was the only instance of intolerance that I showed to my dear wife. (Unp)

After their marriage, Charles and Amélie lived at 35 rue du Faubourg Poissonnière on the third floor of the building that belonged to Amélie's father. Later they moved to 5 rue Bonaparte. Richet did not allow domestic responsibilities to interfere with his customary activities and pleasures. Although he went to the theater frequently with Amélie and occasionally they had guests for dinner, Richet involved himself very little in home life. He spent long periods away from home traveling and writing poetry, novels, and plays. On one such trip in 1879 he completed the translation of Harvey's *De Motu Cordis*.[R 41] When he was in Paris, he often read or wrote in the morning, worked in his laboratory during the afternoon and at night did bibliographic work, often dictating notes to Amélie. In his biographical writing Richet expressed admiration for some of his children's qualities and those of his wife, Amélie, but no sentiment. He wrote that his wife became angry when he told her that after three months at sea on the yacht of Prince Albert of Monaco, the Princesse Alice, none of the passengers knew he was married. "I felt that one should not speak of his wife," he wrote, "It would be pointless to give her great praise."

Alfred described his father's attitude toward his wife as "a sort of veneration" adding, "I think he felt in her elements that were foreign to him, thus constituting a polar attraction. For him she felt an unmitigated and open admiration." Richet's autobiography *Souvenirs d'un Physiologiste* failed altogether to mention his family life or even his wife Amélie except where she was part of a narrative.[R 736] He mentioned but two of his seven children and only as they collaborated in his writings or investigations.

The Death of Sister-in-Law and Mother

In 1883 Amélie's sister Adèle died of a puerperal infection acquired during the birth of her third child. Her doctor, an *agrégé* at the university named Charpentier did not use antisepsis, although it was already well accepted elsewhere in Europe. Richet was outraged and never wanted to see Charpentier again but, as it happened, Richet's mother invited the doctor to dinner. At first Charles refused to join the party but when, "with tears in her eyes," his mother urged him to reconsider, he did. She put her arms around him and said "you are the best of sons." He was glad that he had complied because a few days later his mother left for Carqueiranne where she was killed in an accident. While she was standing near the wall of a dam under construction there, it suddenly collapsed. A huge stone struck and killed her.[1] Some workmen at the base of the wall were also killed by the falling stones. His mother's death was a heavy blow to Charles. The carefree gaiety of his youth, already dampened by the death of his grandfather, was now less evident. For the next ten years, Richet worked harder than ever in his laboratory. He also started teaching a course in physiology at the Ecole Pratique on rue Lhomond with his friend Gley as his assistant.

Election to the Société de Biologie

A prime objective for Richet after achieving his faculty appointment was to present himself as a candidate for election to the Société de Biologie. His wide ranging curiosity and his appetite for synthesis were nourished by the discussions at the meetings of the société which he had attended since his student days. He lost out against Louis Joseph

Landouzy (1845–1917) on his first try and on the second to Albert Jules Franck Dastre (1844–1917).

Shortly thereafter he received a visit from an acquaintance, François Henri Hallopeau (1842–1919) a dermatologist who told Richet that his failure to be elected to the Société de Biologie was unfair and due to the opposition of some powerful people. Hallopeau, already a member, organized a group of friends to support Richet's candidacy; he was elected at the next opportunity. "I was very grateful to Hallopeau for his spontaneous campaign," wrote Richet, "I later supported Hallopeau's bid for appointment to the Faculté de Médecine. It was not only because his competitor did not inspire my interest but mainly because I am not an ingrate" (Unp).

During the years prior to his election to membership Richet had been eager to feel a sense of involvement in the Society. Some of his experiments were suggested by discussions at the regular Saturday afternoon meetings of the Société de Biologie.

Richet treasured his relationship with the Société de Biologie and with the important scientists, including Louis Pasteur, with whom he was privileged to share his ideas. He was particularly fond of the informality of the presentations and the often vigorous and sometimes acrimonious open discussion that followed. The proceedings, which were published monthly, provided Richet with a vehicle with which to establish the priority of his many observations and discoveries without the detailed documentation required by more formal journals.

Research

Lactose as a Diuretic

At a meeting of the Société de Biologie during the presidency of Claude Bernard, a discussion emerged about whether or not internal hemorrhage could be checked by the intravenous injection of milk. Richet, intrigued by the notion, decided to pursue the milk question with his colleague Moutard-Martin. They found, however, that milk injected into the vein of a dog produced only profuse diuresis. After demonstrating that injections of distilled water caused actual cessation of urinary flow, they concluded that the diuretic effect of milk was due to its relatively high concentration of lactose. Subsequently they verified the inference by administering the sugar alone, thus contributing to the later recognition of osmotic diuresis.[R 33]

Others of the topics that Richet selected for his early experiments appeared to have been picked at random but on closer scrutiny one can detect an emerging theme that identifies what was perhaps his most important conceptual contribution to physiology, the idea of "defense of the organism."

That hypothesis finally took shape after his 1887 discovery of passive immunity, (described in chapter 5) but what he learned from his study of the effect of metal salts on bacteria, first published in 1883, may have helped plant the seed of that idea.[R 120]

Working with metallic salts, shown in earlier observations of Raulin to have a lethal effect on cultures of bacteria, (Nid) Richet introduced them in gradually increasing quantity into a culture of lactobacilli in milk. He and his students, Pierre Lasablière, Eudoxie Bachrach, and Henri Cardot, found that this slowly progressive exposure enabled the organisms, through successive generations, to acquire immunity to a normally fatal dose of a metallic salt,[R 78, R 120] clearly indicating genetically regulated adaptation of the bacteria to the metallic poisons.

Adaptive neurological regulatory mechanisms were evident in his studies of summation and refractoriness performed with Antoine Breguet and André Broca, (described in chapter 3). These experiments had intensified his interest in the brain, acquired during his period of internship with Lefort. Likewise his fascination with the pharmacological effects of natural substances was focused on the brain, as evidenced by a monograph he published on the actions of alcohol, chloroform, hashish and coffee, all substances capable of modifying thought and consciousness.[R 38]

Doubtless because of his emerging views about defense of the organism, Richet's curiosity was drawn to questions about the regulation of bodily responses in preference to more conventional inquiries into what organs do or what role they play in the bodily economy. His metabolic and thermoregulatory experiments, described in the next section, were begun shortly before his appointment to the faculty.[R 28] They ultimately showed that the body temperature, although produced by heat generated in living tissues, was regulated in the brain[R 135] and that the mechanism involved could be blocked by anesthetizing the animal. This work culminated in a paper *La Systeme Nerveux et la Chaleur Animale*, which was published at the time of his appointment as professor.[R 208]

The most coherent exposition of his views on defense appears in Richet's chapter, The Functions of Defense in his *Dictionnaire de Physiologie*. In the preamble, he points out that topics that are usually treated as separate, such as nutrition, innervation, and reproduction actually share a common goal, "Their function is to produce appropriate movements or special chemical substances as reactions of defense that can be studied as elements of an all embracing scheme of resistance to a more or less hostile environment (millieu extérieure) and thereby maintain the integrity of the organism."[R 419] He, however, explains that in order to provide necessary details in each case he studied the mechanisms under separate topics such as body heat, heart, phagocytosis, toxicology, diapedesis, pain, and so on, "They must also be considered as an harmonic ensemble of resistance."

Toward the end of the chapter Richet refers to contemporary studies of the glands of internal secretion, the pituitary, adrenal, thyroid, thymus, and kidney that regulate several bodily functions, pointing out how their failure to secrete results in "grave disorders." As he put it, "their products stimulate the nourishment of tissues, restore arterial pressure and enliven the cells of the nervous system. In brief they contribute to the defense of the organism not only by the destruction of poisons, but also by reinforcing the energy of vital functions. Life is a perpetual autoregulation, an adaptation to the changing influences of the environment. The level must perpetually change as it oscillates around a relatively stable mean. In short it reacts to all influences, resisting them and always restoring the original balance."

Metabolic and Thermoregulatory Mechanisms

Now, as *agrégé*, having responsibility for students of his own, Richet was ready to initiate a major research program. He elected to explore further the physiology of metabolic and thermoregulatory mechanisms, the process responsible for "animal heat." It gave him the opportunity to pursue his "defense" idea and to apply his interest in chemistry stimulated by his work in the laboratory of Berthelot. He selected for study the field of his idol, Lavoisier. He found, however, that the laboratory facilities at the Faculté de Médecine were inadequate for his needs. The dean,

Auguste Béclard, therefore assigned him a laboratory in a university building on the Rue Vauquelin.

Laying the background for the study, Richet introduced the subject of his first lecture to the students, tracing the evolution of the thermodynamic theory, beginning with Lavoisier's discovery in 1777 of oxygen consumption during respiration in the animal.[R 132] Next he mentioned a publication issued in 1824, by the French engineer, Nicolas Léonard Sadi Carnot (1796-1832). The English translation, published several years later, "Reflections on the Motive Power of Fire," contained Carnot's early concept that led to the first law of thermodynamics (Carnot 1824). Richet felt that Carnot's contribution had not been given proper credit when, seventeen years later, Julius Von Mayer (1814-1878) proposed the theory (Mayer 1842) which was firmly established in 1847 by Hermann Ludwig Ferdinand von Helmholtz (1821-1894) as the law of the conservation of energy (Helmholtz 1847).

Meanwhile, in 1838, a German physicist, Karl Fredrick Mohr (1806-1879) had put forward the notion of the equivalence of heat and energy and of the transformation of one to the other. Mohr's report was rejected by a major journal; later, when it appeared in an obscure publication, it was ignored (Nid). Credit for the idea was instead assigned to the French engineer, Armand Seguin (1765-1835) who had worked with Lavoisier on respiratory carbon dioxide as an indicator of heat production in animals. Richet included in his lecture an acknowledgement of Dean Béclard's studies of the heat of muscular movement in which he had applied the findings of Antoine Lavoisier.

The above series of developments not only led to the understanding that oxygen was essential to heat production (and hence energy release) and that carbon dioxide and water were the products of the burning or degradation of inanimate objects but that furthermore the same sequence characterized the metabolism of living organisms. The riddle of "animal heat" was thus explained and the long held notion that biological processes differed somehow from inorganic ones by virtue of an added "vital principle" was pretty well dispelled.

A great many investigators had contributed through small steps to the understanding of metabolic combustion and its relationship to breathing. There still remained the question as to whether animal heat was produced in the lungs themselves, the blood, capillaries, or tissues. The ultimate solution to the problem was to some extent predicted in earlier unpublished papers by Lazzaro Spallanzani (1729–1799) who demonstrated respiration in tissues (Spallanzani 1777). Probably unaware of the Spallanzani experiments, Hermann von Helmholtz demonstrated and measured heat produced by the isolated twitch of a frog muscle (Helmholtz 1847). A few years later Claude Bernard passed a catheter through the right auricle of a dog into the hepatic vein. Observing that blood was warmed by passing through the liver, he concluded that metabolic combustion was taking place in that organ. In 1856 he showed that blood was warmed by passage through the wall of the intestines as well, thereby effectively settling the question in favor of local tissue production of the heat of metabolism (Bernard 1856).

Since glucose is a major source of the energy of combustion, Richet reasoned (incorrectly) that if he eliminated sugar from the diet, the process of heat production would be interrupted. He therefore induced tetanic muscular contractions by electrical stimulation in dogs that had been starved for several days. To his surprise he found that their body temperature rose as quickly and as high as did the temperature of similarly stimulated well fed animals. The failure of this experiment enabled Richet to make an important observation. He noted that the elevation of body temperature caused by the electrically induced seizure was accompanied by an acceleration of the animals' panting. He further observed that the body temperature rose even more steeply when the dogs were muzzled and thus unable to open their mouths widely. Richet reasoned that since dogs, lacking sweat glands, cannot, like horses, lose heat through evaporation of sweat, evaporation must take place from the membranes which cover the tongue and line the mouth and respiratory passages of the dog. He further concluded that excessive loss of carbon dioxide is prevented by the shallowness of panting so that, although breathing is rapid, the exchange of air does not reach the depths of the lungs. Richet called this respiratory pattern "polypnea."[R 181] Thus Richet had again turned a failed experiment into a unique fresh observation that enabled him to discover that the brain stem regulates body temperature in dogs by reflex control of the frequency of respiration.

Jean-Paul Langlois, one of Richet's collaborators, added a fascinating observation in comparative neurobiology (Langlois 1906). He found that reflex panting also occurs in cold-blooded vertebrates such as the Sahara lizard. Its rate of respiration was greatly accelerated when the animal was placed in an extremely hot environment. The reflex, by speeding up heat loss through the lizard's respiratory passage, effectively prevented potentially fatal hyperthermia when the lizards were exposed to the sun. Langlois, a man twelve years younger than Richet, became his favorite pupil. Their work together on respiration, anesthesia, body temperature regulation and the distribution of chlorides in the body described in chapter 5 extended from the mid-1880s to the time of Richet's retirement in 1925. Another favorite was Maurice Hanriot (1854–1933) a chemist who was laboratory chief at the Collège Rollin before he joined Richet to collaborate on studies of metabolism. On page 54 of *Souvenirs d'un Physiologiste*, Richet refers to his metabolic work as the one that "in the bottom of my heart I prefer because it provides complete elucidation of a very important point entirely new to physiology. I am amazed that this (the thermoregulatory function of panting in dogs) had never occurred to a physiologist before. What has been demonstrated then is a new function of the brain stem, thermoregulation due to frequency of respiratory movements."[R 736]

Richet's interest in the body's heat production and heat loss had sprung in part from curiosity about how animals keep warm in a cold environment. He recorded the body temperature of dogs, rabbits, birds, and other creatures and found a wide difference in a basal temperature of the various species. He noted that those with the highest body temperature had the richest insulation of fur and feathers. Further, he observed that animals whose natural insulation was insufficient could generate heat by muscle contraction, either voluntarily through exercise, or involuntarily through shivering.

Richet adduced evidence that shivering was triggered by a nervous reflex in response to a cold environment. In a characteristically simple and direct experiment he showed that shivering failed to occur in anesthetized dogs exposed to cold.[R 256] In the absence of shivering there was a sharp decline in body temperature. As soon as the dogs recovered consciousness, however, vigorous shivering began and persisted until the normal temperature was restored.

Cited in Richet's *La Chaleur Animale* is the following historical background for the then current knowledge of the role of the brain in temperature regulation:[R 256] "In 1837 an English surgeon, Sir Benjamin Collins Brodie [1783–1862] had a patient with paraplegia from a cervical spine injury. Forty-two hours before he died his temperature rose to 43.9 degrees C. Later, similar experiences were recorded by Theodor Billroth

[1829-1894], Gustav S. Simon [1824-1876], Heinrich Irenäus Quincke [1842-1922], and others. Naunyn & Quincke confirmed their findings with animal experiments on the medulla, the pons (pont de Varole) and la protuberance annulaire." Richet in 1885 explored the phenomenon and reported his experiments that involved piqure of the brain. He inserted a needle from side to side in a rabbit's head at the level of the anterior region of the orbit. A rapid increase in temperature of two degrees in one hour occurred with no other detectable changes in the animal, except excitability.

Although Richet was not able to state what structures had been impaled by his needle, it is likely from his description of the procedure that it damaged the hypothalamus. Not until 1912, through the experiments of Henry Gray Barbour (1912) and Isenschmid & Krehl (1912), was the hypothalamus clearly shown to be implicated in the regulation and control of body temperature in warm blooded animals.

Richet concluded his monograph *La Chaleur Animale* with these words: "In the final analysis, the nervous system appears to us as the essential agent for animal heat. It directs the chemical activity. It permits the animal to conform to the ambient temperature and to make more or less heat, more or less radiation, more or less evaporation, according to the conditions of the environment."

The year following Richet's piqure experiments, two German medical students Aronsohn and Sachs, working at the laboratory of animal physiology of the Landwirthschaftlichen Hochschule in Berlin, published experiments on the production of fever in animals by destruction of sites in the brain. Their paper, which appeared in *Pflüger's Archiv. für gesammte Physiologie*, failed to acknowledge Richet's priority. In fact, they cited only one non-German language publication, a study by Wood, published in *Smithsonian Contributions* (Aronsohn & Sachs 1886). Richet appealed to Eduard Friedrich Wilhelm Pflüger (1829-1910) to publish a correction. Although Aronsohn and Sachs later acknowledged their oversight, as did Pflüger himself, Pflüger nevertheless refused to publish a correction. "I was a little annoyed" wrote Richet in his *Mémoires*.

In 1886 and 1887 Richet with Hanriot carried out a long series of metabolic experiments on a man named Sauvage who supplied animals to his laboratory. They tested the effects of varying meals on Sauvage's consumption of oxygen, and found that the respiratory quotient, arrived at by dividing the carbon dioxide produced by the oxygen consumed, varied with alimentation; it approached unity after a meal rich in sugar, while during brief periods of fasting it fell toward seventy, but no lower. Altering the depth and frequency of breathing had relatively little effect on gas exchange on the lungs of Sauvage; whatever alterations did occur were quickly corrected.

Sauvage, who had been a willing subject for the seemingly endless metabolic experiments finally failed to appear one day and thereafter never returned. He had been required to subsist on meals of extreme and unappetizing preponderance of protein, carbohydrate or fat, or even on nonfood items such as glycerine. He also had to undergo the discomfort of breathing through the tubes of Richet's instrument for hours on end. When Sauvage no longer appeared at the laboratory and could not be located, he rated from Richet only a casual comment: "then he disappeared without any word and I suppose he died in a hospital."[R 727] Sauvage had, indeed, died of tuberculosis at Hôpital de la Charité as Richet eventually learned from Moutard-Martin who had cared for him there.

Calorimetry

In 1849, Henri Victor Régnault (1810–1878) and Jules Reiset (1818–1896), while pursuing Lavoisier's metabolic discoveries, had constructed a closed system for measuring gas exchange in an animal housed in a glass bell (Régnault 1849). Their design was further extended by Max Joseph Von Pettenkofer (1818–1901) to accommodate the body of a man either lying in bed or working an ergometer (Pettenkofer 1862). Richet built a calorimetric chamber that enabled him to study, not only the consumption of oxygen and the production of carbon dioxide in dogs and other mammals, but also the production and loss of heat.[R 150]

At about the same time Jacques Arsène d'Arsonval (1851–1940) had also developed a calorimeter which he described at a meeting of the Société de Biologie (d'Arsonval 1894). It was built like an egg penetrated by a slender siphon on the principle that the heat of the body should displace the air in the egg which, in turn, would rise to a calibrated reading on the water filled siphon. The device could not record a decrease in body temperature, only an increase above the temperature of the environment. D'Arsonval eventually preferred Richet's design in which the animal was placed in an insulated capsule containing a volatile liquid. Since the heat produced by the animal would volatize the liquid and cause it to escape through the siphon, the height of the displacement should be proportional to the weight of the liquid remaining. With his instrument Richet showed that under basal conditions oxygen consumption varied with the body surface rather than the body mass of the animal. The same discovery had been made entirely independently a few weeks earlier in Germany by Max Rubner (1854–1932) (Rubner 1894) who had also built a metabolic chamber in which temperatures could be measured. Richet summarized his work and that of his predecessors in a monograph published in 1889.[R 256] The summary was also included in a long article in his multi-volume *Dictionnaire de Physiologie*.[R 391]

Again Richet failed to extend very far his groundbreaking contributions. Instead, he left them to be developed by others whose names were eventually accorded more prominence in that field of research than Richet's. Rubner, for example, went on to prove with his apparatus that the law of conservation of energy, formulated by Von Mayer and Helmholtz, applied to the living body. Others including Adolf Magnus-Levy (1865–1955), Graham Lusk (1866–1932), Francis Gans Benedict, (1870–1957) and Eugene Floyd DuBois (1882–1959), made further methodological improvements and advanced our modern understanding of calorimetry. In a comprehensive historical note on respiratory physiology prepared by John F. Perkins for the American Physiological Society's Handbook of Physiology, Richet's name is not even mentioned (Perkins 1964).

Asphyxia And The Dive Reflex

While working in Vulpian's laboratory in 1879 Richet had studied the nervous control of the heartbeat. He applied electrical stimulation to the distal cut end of the vagus nerve and found that the strength of stimulus required to slow or stop the heart was greatly reduced in the presence of oxygen deprivation. The data were not published until fifteen years later when Richet was studying the dive reflex described below.[R 374] This work provided the explanation of the bradycardia (heart rate slowing) known to occur during partial asphyxia.[R 388] Oxygen deprivation was a serious problem for surgeons and physiologists alike because anesthesia with chloroform or morphine suppressed the movements of respiration. Following Richet's demonstration that asphyxia accentuated the vagus nerve's effect of slowing the heartbeat, Paul Bert, who had made classical observations on the physiological effects of variations in atmospheric pressure, described what later became known as the dive reflex. Bert's laboratory was beautifully located near the edge of the Bois de Boulogne in Paris, where a small pond on the grounds was home to a flock of ducks. Bert noted that when the ducks immersed their heads in order to catch fish they were able to hold them under water longer than what he estimated the capacity of their lungs should allow. He therefore held a duck's head under water and made the startling observation that the animal survived up to 10 minutes or more before dying of asphyxia. He also noted that upon immersion there was a remarkable slowing of the duck's heart rate. After confirming his findings, Bert published the observation in 1879, concluding that the duck's relatively large blood volume provided a mechanism for storing oxygen and mobilizing it when needed (Bert 1879).

Charles Richet had noted the possible relevance of Paul Bert's observation on the diving ducks to protection of the organism against asphyxia, but was skeptical of Bert's suggestion that the animals possessed an oxygen storage mechanism. Not until a few years later, however, did Richet challenge Bert's inference experimentally. He found that removal of a large amount of a duck's blood volume did not shorten his survival under water. In other experiments he tied off the tracheas of the ducks. When held under water, some survived as long as twenty minutes. Survival was cut to three to five minutes, however, when their ability to slow their heart rate was prevented by atropine or cutting the vagus nerve. Ducks whose tracheas were tied, but who were not immersed in water also failed to greatly slow their hearts and survived only in the neighborhood of five minutes. Richet concluded that the immersed ducks had actually conserved their supply of oxygen by slowing the circulation of blood to the tissues. He further deduced that the oxygen conserving mechanism was elicited reflexly by water coming into contact with the ducks' heads. He published a short note on the work in 1894. In 1899 he published a more extended report, adding a speculation that the afferent limb of the protective reflex must travel in the trigeminal nerves.[R 416] Richet did not work further to pursue the fascinating and biologically important dive reflex. Indeed, it was almost lost to notice until the 1930s when Laurence Irving (1895–1979) and his students and collaborators embarked on a fruitful investigation of the phenomenon (Irving 1934). Their work extended to the mid 1960s and included such notable investigators as Per Fredrik Scholander (1905–1978) (1962) Harold Torbjorn Andersen (1933–) and others who studied the reflex in a wide variety of birds, reptiles, and mammals. In addition to the slowing of the heart rate, they found a powerful arterial constriction in skin, muscles and in internal organs except for the brain.

By a series of nerve-cutting experiments Andersen established that the reflex depended on the integrity of the ophthalmic branch of the trigeminal nerve, thereby confirming Richet's earlier speculation (Andersen 1963). Eugene Debs Robin (1919–) and Hershel Victor Murdaugh, Jr. (1928–) studying oxygen consumption in harbor seals following a dive, found that the apneic period (the period of breath holding under water) was not compensated for by a proportional increase in oxygen consumption on emergence from the water, so that only 50 percent of the accumulated oxygen debt was repaid (Robin & Murdaugh 1963). Victor Pachon, one of Richet's brightest students, had already reported in 1907 that oxygen demand as well as oxygen consumption was immediately reduced on immersion of ducks in water (Pachon 1907), a discovery Robin and Murdaugh failed to cite.

Scholander and associates demonstrated the diving reflex in man. His studies of Japanese pearl divers showed that they not only slowed their heart rate, but displayed a variety of disturbances of cardiac rhythm as well. L. Stanley James found the diving reflex to be present in the human fetus immersed in amniotic fluid prior to birth (James 1958). He was able to correlate the degree of heart rate slowing (bradycardia) and increase in lactic acid in umbilical cord blood with the extent of fetal distress during the first stage of labor. Robert Elsner (1920–) and Brett Gooden (1943–) showed that the reflex was not only phylogenetically ancient, but was also dominant when competitive with other protective reflex mechanisms, such as enhancement of blood flow to a limb during exercise or after a period in which the circulation was interrupted (Elsner & Gooden 1970). In fishes the reflex was found to be elicited by removal from the water, their normal source of oxygen. Even in marine invertebrates low on the phylogenetic scale, such as the sea slug, aplysia, prompt slowing of heart rate occurred when the animal was removed from the water (Feinstein 1977). Richet had thus opened an important field of study involving a protective reflex that was not only phylogenetically ancient but predominant over other potentially competing adaptive mechanisms that had evolved more recently.

Chesterfield Garvan Gunn (1920–) found that an electrical stimulus applied at a single site in the brain near the nucleus of the tractus solitarius would produce all the features of the dive reflex without immersion of the face in water. The nucleus of the tractus solitarius is responsive not only to stimuli from the environment, but to emotionally activated circuits in the forebrain as well (Gunn 1972). Further studies showed that the dive reflex in man is greatly enhanced during anxiety and fear, but is inhibited during preoccupation and mental concentration (Wolf 1965), observations that would have greatly interested Richet.

Editorial, Literary, Historical, and Bibliographic Work

In 1881, only three years after his appointment to the Faculté de Médecine, Richet was asked to become editor-in-chief of *La Revue des Cours Scientifique*, later called *Revue Scientifique*, a semipopular journal, the contents of which was intended to be intelligible to educated laymen as well as scientists. It was known colloquially as *La Revue Rose*. Since Richet was weak in mathematics and felt inadequate to judge papers that involved complex mathematical interpretations, he persuaded his friend Antoine Breguet, now a widely respected engineer and associate of Marey, to join him as associate editor. Richet immersed himself in this journalistic undertaking with great enthusiasm. He enjoyed immensely his work as an editor and, according to his grandson, Gabriel, he was as enthusiastic about journalism as about science.

Richet, also hoping to combine fishing with science, spent 12,000 francs to build an aquarium on a small inlet near Carqueiranne. He learned very little physiology at the aquarium but found it an ideal setting for writing. Two nonmedical pieces created there were an essay, "A la Recherche de la Gloire" (Nid) and a novel *Une Conscience d'Homme* (Nid).

In 1882 Charles and Amélie moved from 5 rue Bonaparte to an apartment at 15 rue de l'Université, a building owned by his father, where Richet's sister Louise lived with her husband Charles Buloz, the editor of the fashionable journal *Revue des Deux Mondes*. Richet acquired a financial interest in the journal which published the work of leading authors in France and elsewhere in Europe. Every Tuesday evening

Charles and Amélie attended a meeting of the editorial board at his sister's apartment which served as the office for the *Revue*. The journal soon became a favored repository for Richet's own prose and poetry.[2] It also served as a vehicle for the publication of reports on his experiences with metapsychology. One novel about the occult that appeared in the *Revue des Deux Mondes* was called *Possession*.[R 220] His friend Octave Houdaille like it so much that he made it into a play and had it produced at la Potinière Theatre.

The Science of Metapsychology

Quoting from *Le Savant*, "The scientific spirit is curiosity," Richet's student and friend, André Mayer (1875-1959) contended that Richet's interest in psychology was entirely consistent with his commitment to medical science (Mayer 1936). He further suggested that Richet's views on psychology may have been shaped by the intellectual atmosphere of his youth when the works of Condillac and Tracy evoked the promise of one day explaining psychological phenomena, thoughts, desires and intelligence in physical terms of the machinery of the brain.

For Richet the strange achievements of mediums, including clairvoyance, the ability to move objects without touching them and the ability to make human forms materialize, were aspects of a special capability of certain people with specialized brains. He believed, therefore, that such phenomena should be considered as part of psychology and hence of physiology to be studied by experiment as should any unexplained phenomenon. To classify such strange occurrences Richet invented the term *métapsychique* from the Greek meaning "beyond the soul." The term has appeared in English translation as metapsychology.

Richet believed that, as chemistry had emerged from alchemy, a new science of the mind would emerge from metapsychology. He persuaded his friend, Jean Meyer, a wealthy industrialist, who had founded a society for the propagation of spiritualism, to establish a society for "the impartial scientific investigation of psychical phenomena." It was formed in 1919 as the Institut Métapsychique.

Richet was not alone among prominent physicians, scientists and philosophers in his penchant for the serious study of strange psychical phenomena. Among those who shared his curiosity and enthusiasm were Pierre Janet (1859-1947) a pupil of Charcot, who later was appointed professor of experimental and comparative psychology at the Collège de France. Others included such distinguished figures as the physical chemist Sir William Crookes (1832-1919) the discoverer of thallium and inventor of the cathode ray tube; Pierre (1859-1906) and Marie (1867-1934) Curie (both of whom had won the Nobel Prize); the English physicist Sir Oliver Lodge (1851-1940), the French philosopher Henri Bergson (1859-1941), the American philosopher William James, the German philosopher and biologist Hans Diersche, the German psychiatrist Baron Von Schrenk-Notzing and the Italian physician-criminologist Cesare Lombroso (1836-1909). Lord Arthur James Balfour (1848-1930), also an enthusiastic member of Great Britain's Society for Psychical Research, became sort of patron of the "believers" among whom were his sister Mildred, principal of Newnham College at Cambridge and wife of moral philosophy professor of Trinity College, Henry Sidgwick. Richet was welcomed into the society and in 1905 became its president.

Experiences with Psychics

Richet was convinced that the seemingly impossible feats of spiritualists were not supernatural but obeyed natural laws not yet familiar to us. With his fascination with Greek, he coined new terms for each accomplishment, cryptesthesia for clairvoyance, telekinesis for unexplained movements and ectoplasm for emanations. In 1885, with the Russian scientist Alexander Asakov, Imperial Councillor to the Czar of Russia, Cesare Lombroso, the astronomer Giovanni Schiaparelli and two other friends, Richet visited Milan to participate in experiments with the notorious medium, Eusapia Palladino. He was so impressed that he brought Eusapia to France where she held seances that were attended by many of Richet's friends including Sarah Bernhardt, the Curies, Frederic Myers, Schrenk-Notzing and Pierre Janet. Eusapia was later exposed as a fraud by a committee of scientists who had visited her in Naples; they published their report in the *Society for Psychical Research Proceedings* (Fielding 1909). Despite the exposé many of the faithful continued to believe that much of her performance was authentic. Richet, himself was convinced that during a session held by another medium, Marthe Béreaud, at the Villa Carmen in Algiers, he had seen an authentic effusion of ectoplasm. Richet required Ben-Boa, the "person" who materialized, to breathe into an aqueous solution of barium hydroxide and thereby demonstrated the presence of carbon dioxide in his breath. On another occasion, at the Institut Métapsychique, Richet had secretly mixed cholesterin in with the paraffin with which a cast of the materialized spirit would be made in order to head off the possibility of fraud by the substitution of a previously prepared cast. Finding cholesterin in the cast further strengthened his conviction of authenticity.

In 1885 Richet helped found the Société de Psychologie Physiologique. Charcot was made president. Pierre Janet and Théodule Ribot (1839–1916) were made vice presidents and Richet, secretary. According to Wundt, "Charcot for years remained a stranger to its deliberations and therefore had little to do with its activities' (Wundt 1893).Richet arranged the first general meeting of the Société in 1889 at the restaurant of the Eiffel Tower, recently erected for the world exposition in Paris. It was attended by psychologists, philosophers, men of letters, and métapsychics but Charcot, the president, possibly wishing to distance himself from Richet's *Métapsychique*, had refused to attend, but nevertheless had dinner in another part of the restaurant. Richet took over the leadership and made the gathering a great success. The second meeting of the Société was held in 1890 in Munich, having been organized by Schrenk-Notzing. That year Richet was approached by a physician named Darrieux who suggested that he and Richet establish a journal concerned with psychic science. Of Darrieux, Richet wrote, "He was a small man, thin, timid, hesitant and lacking in charm. After some hesitation I agreed and we founded *Annales des Sciences Psychiques* which later became known as *Revue Métapsychique*" (Unp). It was in constant financial difficulty. Richet's friend Eugene Osty, director of the Institut Métapsychique International tried to keep it alive but after his death in 1938 and then the start of the second World War the journal ceased publication in 1940 (Mauskopf & McVaugh 1980). The Society has persisted, however, with its headquarters in Paris at 1 Place Wagram. Dr. Hubert Larcher is the current director.

In 1886 Richet propounded his theory of the unconscious. It appeared in a festschrift for Michel Eugène Chevreul (1786–1889). Chevreul, a pioneer organic and industrial chemist,had published in 1854 an essay on table turning and other extraordinary feats of spiritualists. Richet's paper attempted to explain the phenomena in physiological terms as due to movements made unconsciously. He inferred the existence of two types of intellectual phenomena, conscious and unconscious. "All powers considered supernatural are but human powers, muscular or psychic," he wrote, "but since they are removed from awareness they appear to have arisen from outside ourselves."[R 190]

"I am well aware," continued Richet, "that a sort of legend has grown up around me and that I have been accused of being a spiritualist inclined toward mysticism. The reverse is true. I have sought a simple, rational and physiological explanation of the phenomena on which spiritualists have based their doctrine. The interpretation I made in 1886 [concerning unconscious behavior] has since been repeatedly confirmed in numerous researches." There were other workers as well who, prior to Freud, had called attention to activities of an individual that may proceed without awareness. Freud finally formulated the notion and documented the fact that such an unconscious process may affect a person's behavior even though he cannot report on it. William James, who opposed much of Freud's psychodynamic theory and his therapeutic methods, nevertheless declared that Freud's insight concerning the unconscious was the most important step forward in his time (Whyte 1962). James, who shared many of Richet's ideas about psychic phenomena, became co-founder of the American Society for Psychical Research.

In 1887 Richet published his *Essai de Psychologie Générale*, a book that was intended to link physiology and psychology as aspects of the same science, that of the brain which controls visceral functions as well as attitudes, emotions, thoughts and behavior. Most of the text had been written at Carqueiranne where he and his children, from whom he had acquired a case of whooping cough, were recuperating. With a phylogenetic approach he attempted to show how a "reflex center becomes an intellectual center." This was an important concept, not necessarily original with Richet, but nevertheless opposed to the views of the influential British physiologist-physician, Marshall Hall (1790–1857) whose book published in 1832, ON THE REFLEX FUNCTION OF THE MEDULLA OBLONGATA AND THE MEDULLA SPINALIS caused him to be identified as the originator of the reflex theory (Hall 1832). Hall considered the neural mechanisms responsible for such automatic reactions to be entirely separate from mechanisms that serve voluntary or emotionally engendered responses of the body. Richet, on the other hand, held that they were at opposite ends of a continuum in a range of complexity that involved the same nervous connections. In chapters dealing with irritability of cells, reflex and instinctive functions, awareness, perception, memory, imagination, and will, Richet described the mechanics of the brain as the mechanics of the person. The book was immensely successful, ran to ten editions, and was translated into Italian, Russian, Hungarian and Polish.

An Important Promotion and a Party to Celebrate Richet's Triumph

After Jules Béclard's death in 1887 no one appeared to compete with Richet for the chair of physiology. Paul Camille Hippolyte Brouardel (1837-1906) who had succeeded Beclard as dean, had mentioned to Richet that the distinguished Chauveau had seemed to consider applying for the post and had commented: "The Chair of Physiology at the Faculté de Médecine is *Ce qu'il y a de plus beau au monde.*"[3] Brouardel made no reply and Chauveau did not submit his name. Richet was appointed to the chair of physiology without opponents. He reacted to his good fortune with the same casual satisfaction with which he accepted his wealth, position, and usual good luck.

Upon his advancement to professor, a group of friends of his youth, Henri Ferrari, Gustave and Paul Ollendorf, Paul and Gaston Fournier, and Roger Alexandre, together with Louis Olivier, Emile Gley, and Paul Langlois, hosted a banquet at the Hôtel Continental on 15 November 1887. The day before the banquet a fire broke out in Richet's laboratory in the rue Vauquelin. Everything was destroyed, including a collection of congratulatory letters that Richet had saved for the occasion. During the night before the fire, two of his colleagues, Ferrari and Héricourt had both dreamed of fire and flames. On the day of the fire and before its discovery, Léonie Boulanger, a medium in Le Havre, with whom Richet and Pierre Janet shared experiences of clairvoyance, told Janet, who had invited her to the celebration, "It is burning, it is burning." Richet recounted the episode in his *Mémoires* as a convincing incident of premonition. Thanks to dean Béclard, the loss was not catastrophic. Richet had a brand new laboratory awaiting him at the medical school. He appointed Paul Langlois laboratory chief and Jules Héricourt assistant chief. There, with Hanriot who became chief of the chemical division, Richet concluded his experimental study of respiration.

Only nineteen years had passed since Richet's enrollment at the Faculté de Médecine. Among the letters of congratulations he received after the banquet was one from Louis Pasteur in which he wrote, "Your speech at the banquet was most charming. If your lively intelligence continues faithful to its inspirations, to love of homeland, you will do great things."

Notes

1. Mme.Gerard de Montebello, a cousin and close friend of Richet's mother, Adèle, told Charles of a premonition of his mother's violent death. At the house of a friend Mme. de Montebello had encountered a medium who had told her that "someone dear to her would die in a horrible accident, crushed by wall falling on her." Richet wrote that his mother's death occurred a few weeks later.
2. The *Revue des Deux Mondes* had been launched as a journal of culture for the intelligents by Buloz' grandfather in 1831. The high quality of its contents had earned it a broad international following. Charles Buloz had become editor in 1869 and continued until 1893, when he became involved in a scandal described in chapter 5.
3. The best in the world.

5

The Young Professor 1887–1902

Richet became professor at thirty-seven, a very young age for his day and an achievement that gave great satisfaction to his father, Alfred, whose influence in furthering his son's career was certainly not inconsiderable.

Young Richet had grown to manhood during the relatively affluent early days of the Third Republic, blessed with wealth and social influence. He was additionally fortunate to have been promoted to the chair of physiology at a time when France had begun to commit significant financial support to medical science in the universities. Thereby he was able to take full advantage of his position, managing to increase his research space and obtain outside financial support, even from the municipal government of Paris.

Richet revelled in his duties as professor and held the post until his retirement thirty-eight years later. One of his students, André Mayer described Richet as "a very striking figure of remarkable vitality, tall, thin and agile with sudden angular gestures that were nevertheless elegant. He spoke to his classes with his head held high looking over the heads of the students. His voice was vibrant and emphatic. He spoke at times with enthusiasm, at others roguishly and sometimes as if lost in a dream" (Mayer 1936).

Richet's *Leçon Inaugurale*, his first lecture as professor began with a statement that was altogether inconsistent with his characteristically wide ranging interests, activities and commitments: "The day the professors of the faculty of medicine of Paris honored me with the chair of physiology, the goal of my life had been achieved. I assure you that this is a commitment almost awesome, to consecrate my entire life to teaching and to science." He went on to review the history of physiology at the university, pointing out that there had been no teaching of physiology throughout the sixteenth and seventeenth centuries and that in the eighteenth-century the professors had offered only vague commentaries on the writings of Hippocrates and Galen, while ignoring the experimental contributions of Harvey and Haller.

As Richet recounted, the first holder of the chair of physiology at Paris was François Chaussier appointed in 1795.[1] Auguste Henri Dumeril (1812–1870) succeeded to the chair in 1831 and after him Pierre Bérard was appointed. François-Achille Longet (1811–1871) succeeded to the chair in 1853 when, thanks to the work of Magendie and Claude Bernard, physiology in France had become independent of anatomy. Richet, who considered him "the first truly experimental professor," recounted how at the meetings of the Société de Biologie, Longet frequently disputed with Magendie and Claude Bernard on a variety of subjects. According to Richet this rivalry was productive, enhancing the contributions of all three. Longet served until 1872 when he was succeeded by Auguste Béclard, the immediate predecessor of Charles Richet.

Richet's lecture emphasized the importance of physics and chemistry to physiology and furthermore that medicine itself is an extension of physiology. Like Rudolph Ludwig Karl Virchow (1821–1902), Richet considered physiology as a social as well as a biological science. Moreover he believed that science in general and physiology in particular would be the means of enhancing the quality of human life and mitigating human suffering. His lecture concluded with a prescription for the practicing physician: "apart from the mission to treat the sick, he should understand the natural history of diseases and should carefully judge conventional practices and popular remedies. In short, the physician should exercise the curiosity of a scholar-scientist without compromising the welfare of his patient."[R 237]

Richet sent a copy of his first lecture to Pasteur who acknowledged it as follows: "Dear Professor, It was with lively emotion that I read of the [possible benefits] of physiology granted a long life, what beautiful discoveries could you not dream of as you remain faithful to experimentation. L. Pasteur." Despite Pasteur's admonition and despite his almost monastic vow in his *Leçon Inaugurale*, Richet found it difficult to devoutly practice the religion of science as a model savant. He could bring himself to practice it only part time, continuing to be susceptible to distraction from his research by his historical interests, his poetry, novels and plays, or by social concerns such as eugenics, the defense of peace, of Dreyfus,[2] of Esperanto or of metapsychology. Travel and entertainment also continued to intrude on his time for the laboratory. Despite his social sophistication, his broad education and experience, Richet might fairly be characterized as naive and as maintaining the conflicting attitudes of adolescence. In my long interview with his son, Alfred, then ninety-four years old, the contradictions in Richet's personality became evident. His vanity, egotism, intolerance and scorn of lesser men, as expressed in his attitude toward lower classes and colored races, his commitment to eugenics, were balanced by his deep sense of propriety, his lack of guile, his loyalty, steadfastness and courage as reflected in his behavior during the scandal described later in this chapter involving his sister's husband, and his remarkable valor during the First World War. In essence Richet was an intellectual with limitless curiosity who felt responsible for maintaining and advancing the noble qualities of man and the glory of France.

Alfred remembered his father being away from home a great deal, often traveling abroad. Alfred added that his father never gave up his lighthearted devotion to his friends and to the games, sports, and the insouciant pleasures he enjoyed with them. He loved roulette at Monte Carlo and often won a great deal with his Martingale strategy (doubling the bet when he lost). "These," said Alfred, "were his little games; his big games were to challenge the 'impossible,' like his attempt to achieve powered flight. In his physiological research he did not go deeply enough into his discoveries. He was content with a sketchy picture. To use a military term, my father did not exploit his successes. An exception was his work on anaphylaxis which he pursued with intensity and in considerable depth."

When at home in Paris Richet played whist or bridge every evening after dinner. At Carqueiranne his evenings were devoted to playing billiards or to teaching his children to play checkers. It was chiefly at Carqueiranne and le Ribaud that Richet was able to spend time with his children. As Alfred put it, his father's relationship with his children was, "alternately playful and imperious, but always with high expectations. To me he was like a king. I trembled when at dinner he asked 'what grade did you get on your last composition?'" Of fishing trips with his father in the waters around le Ribaud Alfred wrote in a letter to his son, Denis: "At 5 A.M., alone in the boat with him on the way to the fishing spot he made me translate Virgil or Tacitus.[3] I resented his comments on the compositions I was required to write for him every day, but without ever doubting his love. In my desire to identify with him without losing my individuality I longed for discussion of a religious topic. His wish to separate his children after their adolescence from Catholic beliefs and practices caused inner conflict for my brother Albert and me."

The Death of Richet's Father

Prior to 1870, to ease the burden of his very successful private practice and to seek a little relaxation from the pressures of work at the university, Richet's father bought a property in Epinay, a rural community east of Paris. Shortly thereafter, the Franco-Prussian War forced him back into full-time service as a military surgeon working day and night. After the war he was rewarded with an appointment as Commandeur de la Légion d'Honneur but he found that Epinay had been all but destroyed by the Prussians. Disillusioned, in 1873 he bought a château with a surrounding farm on the Mediterranean coast of southern France at Carqueiranne and gave the Epinay property to his daughter Louise.

Shortly after Charles' appointment as professor, his father having by then dominated French surgery for twenty-five years, retired and spent most of the year at Carqueiranne. At retirement he was reputed to have made the remarkable statement that he had produced only two things in his life "mon fils et mon livre," my son and my book. Four years later in 1891 Alfred died of pneumonia. He had gone to Carqueiranne to spend the winter feeling well and, as Charles expressed it, "having bright eyes," when he suddenly developed an upper respiratory infection with bronchitis and symptoms of flu which developed into bronchopneumonia. Charles received a telegram calling him to his father's bedside. "Already," wrote Richet, "candidates hoping to succeed to his seat at the Institut were swarming, especially their wives." Charles arrived at Carqueiranne and examined his father's chest but found little. That night Alfred became delirious. Charles wired his sister to come and within a few days Alfred was dead.

At his father's death, Charles inherited a considerable fortune, including the château at Carqueiranne with its large and profitable surrounding farm property. Now, a professor facing few teaching requirements apart from occasional lectures, he spent more and more time in Carqueiranne fishing and writing.

The house at 15 rue de l'Université was divided between Charles and his sister Louise. Her husband, Charles Buloz, editor-in-chief of *Revue des Deux Mondes* in which Richet and Louise had financial interest, hesitated to share the house at first but a satisfactory division was worked out with separate interior staircases.

Richet set about designing a library that resembled that of Charcot. The walls were lined with two tiers of book shelves, the upper level being accessed by a spiral staircase and lighted from the ceiling. In addition to his own books which he bought in profusion from dealers all over France and his grandfather Renouard's classical library, the collection included the surgery books and a valuable collection of theses from his father's library, literary volumes given to him by his uncle Casimir Chevreux, an uniquely complete collection of "Bulletins de la Société de Biologie and series of various other journals. His library became Charles Richet's most prized possession." "I think," he wrote, "that it gives an aesthetic impression of peace and of work. The portraits of my father, my grandfather and my great grandfather hang there to indicate that perhaps a part of them still watches over their boy."

Richet's Students and Collaborators

Most of Richet's collaborators were friends and associates near his own age. Some of them, as private practitioners, had access to populations of patients. Richet had hoped his laboratory would become a *foyer intellectuel* for young medical scientists, a launching pad, as it were, for brilliant young people. However, Richet's contacts with his students were continually interrupted for literary, editorial, political and other distractions. Only a minority of the medical students registered for a science degree in addition to the M.D. and many of those who did gravitated toward other professors who were more or less constantly available in their own laboratories.

Despite the limited number of students, Richet nevertheless attracted several talented young people who later gained prominence. Among them were Victor Pachon, who became director of the Institut Marey and later professor of physiology at Bordeaux; Emile Abelous, who became professor and eventually dean at Toulouse; Paul Langlois; Emile Bardier; who followed Abelous as professor at Toulouse; Jean Athanasiu (1868–1926) a Rumanian who became professor of physiology at Bucharest,

and Mariette Pompillian, also a Rumanian. Athanasiu who, after completing his training with Richet, wanted to marry Pompillian, offered her
a faculty post in Bucharest. She declined, having decided to turn her
interests to art and music and become a French citizen. Another outstanding pupil was Joachim Carvallo, a young Spaniard who joined Richet in
1893. Richet had learned of Carvallo from a colleague, R. Calderon
Yarena, whom he had met while working in Berthelot's laboratory.
Richet, noting that Carvallo appeared undernourished, arranged for him
to live with Victor Pachon, another relatively impecunious student,
sharing the cost of rent so that both would have more funds available for
food.

Richet was conscientious about promoting the careers of those few
doctoral and postdoctoral students that he had by sending them to other
laboratories to enlarge their experience, Pachon to Marey for example.
He sent another student, Lucien Bull, to America to work on calorimetry
with Francis G. Benedict (1870–1957), successor to Wilbur O. Atwater
(1844–1907) at the Carnegie Institution of Washington. Bull had been
working with Mariette Pompillian trying to develop an improved calorimeter for metabolic studies. Richet appointed Athanasiu, Pachon and
Carvallo in sequence as directors of Paul Bert's old laboratory in the Bois
de Boulogne, which became the Institut Marey.

As prominent as some of his students became, however, Richet failed
to establish a "school" for young physiologists as Pasteur and Bernard
had. Claude Bernard's former students, Paul Bert and d'Arsonval used
the word "paternal" to describe their chief's attitude to themselves.
According to Paul Bert, Bernard on his deathbed addressed his pupils as
his "scientific family." Bert added that Bernard's affection for his students never led him to be indulgent of their weaknesses: "Although
generous with praise and encouragement, he was as sternly critical of the
work of his associates as of his own" (Bert 1879).

If Richet had a paternal feeling for any of his students it would
probably be Joachim Carvallo whose brilliance, resourcefulness and
broad relationship to life resembled to some extent the career of Richet.

Richet delegated the further pursuit of his research on the stomach to
Carvallo who began by collaborating with Pachon.[4] They added important new information to Richet's earlier findings. While exploring the
consequences of life without a stomach they succeeded in performing
the world's first successful gastrectomy on an animal. Carvallo described

the feat in his extensive review of research on the stomach in Richet's *Dictionnaire de Physiologie*: "Discouraged by our fruitless attempts to completely remove a dog's stomach, and wishing to ascertain whether or not life was possible without a stomach, we switched experimental subjects in order to achieve our goal" (Carvallo 1902). They found a cat to be suitable to their objective and, on 4 November 1894, managed a successful removal of a cat's stomach. They named the animal Agastre (without a stomach). Not only did the cat survive but, after a few weeks of recovery, ate well and gained weight. Soon thereafter, however, the cat seemed to lose all interest in food. Carvallo and Pachon concluded that the stomach itself might contain sensory structures important to hunger and appetite. Carvallo tube fed the animal for a time and the cat did well, but ultimately Carvallo gave up and the cat died six months after the operation. At autopsy, "there was no trace of lesions in any of the organs."[5]

In one respect Joachim Carvallo's approach to life differed sharply from that of Richet. In contrast to his mentor's neutral attitude toward marriage Carvallo actually fell in love. The object of his attention was a fellow student for whom Richet had, perhaps, his deepest personal attachment, Anna Coleman. Anna was a wealthy young American woman who came to study in Richet's laboratory in 1879. Carvallo pursued her despite the fact that the war between Spain and the United States that was taking place at the time sparked heated exchanges between them. Anna eventually rejected Carvallo's advances, cut short her period of study in Paris and returned home to her family in Lebanon, Pennsylvania. Richet accepted her abandonment of physiology because, although she had been highly conscientious and dependable, he considered her a poor experimenter. "Physiology was not her vocation," he wrote. Richet kept in touch with her nevertheless and made a side trip to Lebanon to see her during his visit to Montreal for a meeting of the British Medical Association.

Carvallo, undaunted, continued to press his suit and showered Anna with letters. Two years later, in exasperation, she returned to Paris to reject in person his unwanted pursuit. Carvallo apparently supplemented his earlier correspondence with effective persuasion since within two weeks of her return to Paris she and Carvallo appeared at Richet's laboratory announcing plans to be married. The wedding took place in December 1899.

Carvallo continued his research on the stomach with enterprise, imagination and freshness of approach comparable to that of his chief. Fascinated by Walter Cannon's recently published X-ray pictures of the stomach in various stages of contraction and relaxation,[6] Carvallo created a device capable of displaying the contractions of the stomach in motion. His invention was based on the principle of Marey's "fusil photographique" with which Marey had studied the aerodynamics of the flight of birds. Its construction was similar to that of the British gatling gun in which bullets could be fired rapidly from a rotating chamber. Marey used photographic film on a rotating disc and thereby developed what was probably the first motion picture camera. Carvallo attached his instrument to an X-ray tube, thus enabling him to make the first visual recordings of gastric motility and thereby to anticipate the development of the fluoroscope. The work became the topic of his thesis for the MD degree.

Carvallo did very little further research although Richet had appointed him to succeed Victor Pachon as director of the Institut Marey. By 1902 Carvallo had begun collecting paintings and other art works and in 1907 he resigned as director of the Institute Marey. As his interests strayed from physiology, his thesis remained unpublished until 1911 (Carvallo 1911). After his resignation from the Institut Carvallo announced to Richet that, "with great reluctance," he was leaving physiology because the previous year he and Anna had purchased the magnificent Château de Villandry in Touraine in the Loire Valley and would have to devote their full time to restoring it. According to Carvallo's grandson, Robert, Anna had wanted a place in the country where she and her husband could do research. He, however, wanted a place to hang his paintings. The chateau had been built in the sixteenth-century by Jean-le Breton, secretary of state under King François I.

The task of repair and remodeling the château proved to be a severe financial strain, even for the wealthy Anna.[7] Carvallo, however, was able to effect the passage of the French government of the "Demeures Historiques," a series of laws that partly excuse from taxation private homes of historical and cultural significance to the nation. The new laws also provided governmental subsidy for major repairs to the buildings. They required the owners to open part of their property to the public but allowed them to retain the admission fees. Dr. and Mrs. Carvallo must, therefore, be given major credit for the survival of the magnificent chateaux of France and for their accessibility to visitors. Dr. Carvallo died in 1936. His wife Anna continued to live at the chateau until her death in 1941. Villandry now belongs to Robert Carvallo, grandson of Joachim.

Although Richet could readily understand Carvallo's independent spirit as well as his interest in aesthetics, he criticized his former student, not for abandoning physiology, but for having "changed radically after his marriage from a democratic socialist free thinker to a committed Catholic monarchist who read only St. Thomas Aquinas and St. Augustine having tasted of science and hence having accepted the authority of reason, to return to popular Christian beliefs or Mohamedan or Buddhist (because they are all the same) puzzles me." He added, "I can only concede the miracle, that my excellent friend Carvallo has been touched by grace" (Unp.). Anna, who was a Protestant, had converted to Catholicism and became deeply involved in religion. (In later life, having studied the Bible in Greek and seeking deeper spiritual satisfaction, she learned Hebrew).

Despite his disappointment over their changed beliefs Richet continued his friendship with the Carvallos, corresponding with them and visiting them at their château. Carvallo's grandson Robert and Gabriel Richet continue the family friendship.

Associations in Britain and Canada

Richet attended a meeting of the British Association for Science in 1898 in Toronto, Canada. He had been invited to be the guest of William Osler who was staying in a house a few miles from town. Upon arriving in Toronto by train from New York, Richet took a coach to the address given him. The coachman dropped him with his luggage at No. 13 on the correct street. It was nearing midnight and raining heavily. After the coachman had left, Richet found the gate locked. There was no response to his ring. "I decided to ring furiously," he wrote in his *Mémoires*. Very soon Osler appeared at the door of No. 15 and welcomed the dripping Richet into the house where he was awaiting him with John Shaw Billings (1839–1913) who, like Osler, was a member of the original Johns Hopkins faculty. Later Billings founded the first great medical library in America, now known as the National Library of Medicine. Also awaiting Richet was Michael Foster (1836–1907) professor of physiology at

Cambridge University in England and biographer of Claude Bernard (Foster 1899). "Excellent Foster," wrote Richet, "classical physiologist, finest of men who was without his pipe as rarely as I." Later Richet met Foster under more difficult circumstances at a subsequent meeting of the British Association for Science in Dover. The British were exasperated by the news of the second conviction of Dreyfus and many among them refused to associate with their French colleagues. Richet was able to reassure Foster, who was president of the association, that he and his colleagues were also outraged. In fact, Louis Edward Grimaux, (1835–1900) a chemist who was president of the French Association, was a strong supporter of Dreyfus.

Research

The work in Richet's laboratory was not confined to physiology. As he wrote in his *Mémoires*, "Although a laboratory of physiology was required, I was resolved not to limit myself to physiology, but also to extend myself into experimental pathology."

Bromides in Epilepsy

From the days when he was studying Marcellin's gastric juice in the laboratory of Berthelot at the Collège de France, Richet had been curious about the significance of the ubiquitous chloride in the body. At that time he had tried, by feeding bromides to dogs, to induce their stomachs to secrete hydrobromic instead of hydrochloric acid. He was unsuccessful but remained intrigued by the possibility. An opportunity to study chloride replacement by bromide arrived with the development of new methods of chemical analysis that allowed for the study of urinary excretion of chloride. As noted earlier, Richet had found that the kidney adjusts the quantity of salt it excretes, depending on the salt content of the diet. By analyzing tissues removed at autopsy from animals that had consumed diets extremely high or low in sodium chloride, Richet learned that the tissue chloride concentration had remained almost constant despite large differences in diet. From this Richet concluded that the body has an avidity for halogens (chlorine, bromine, fluorine) and must maintain a certain concentration of them in the blood and tissues.

Recalling his earlier experiment in which he failed to induce the stomach to secrete bromides by adding them to the diet of his dogs, he reasoned that cells must have a greater affinity for chloride than for bromide.[8] Based on these considerations he conceived of a way to improve on the potassium bromide treatment of epilepsy.

Clinicians at that time were prescribing very large doses of potassium bromide to control epileptic seizures. In the hope of reducing the effective dose, Richet proposed to a clinical colleague a psychiatrist named Edouard Toulouse (1865–1947), that epileptic patients be treated by sharply reducing their intake of sodium chloride. He reasoned that if the bromides should replace the chloride in the tissues, a much smaller dose of potassium bromide than previously required might control their epileptic seizures. The happy outcome was that Toulouse was able to control seizures with an average dose of bromides reduced from twelve to two grams daily. On the strength of their success Richet devised a name for the treatment "the metatrophic method," a term that failed to become popular among physicians.

Richet continued his study of the control of distribution of chlorides in the body with Langlois. They showed that normally the concentration of chloride in the body is unaffected by salt loading or deprivation. The work led to the discovery of the cause of edema, the abnormal retention of sodium chloride in the body thus anticipating the discoveries of Fernand Widal (1862–1929) in Paris and Hermann Strauss (1808–1944) in Berlin in which a primary role was assigned the chloride ion (Widal 1905) (Strauss, 1903).

Chloralose—to Block Pain

Another chemical challenge that intrigued Richet was the possibility of safely immobilizing animals during experiments that required vivisection and at the same time blocking pain sensation. Curare, which paralyzes the animals but does not relieve pain, was most widely used at the time. Some investigators added chloroform anesthesia but it was generally considered unsatisfactory because it suppressed respiration and hence often produced fatal oxygen lack. Although ether had been used in the United States for surgical anesthesia since the famous Massachusetts General Hospital demonstration in 1847, it was not much used in Europe for animal experimentation. England's most prominent neurophysiologist Charles Scott Sherrington (1856-1952) used decerebration, surgically isolating the pain sensitive areas from the rest of the brain, in preference to anesthesia so as to avoid suppressing the neural circuitry under study.

Although throughout his scientific career Richet was criticized by animal welfare groups for performing vivisection, he was nevertheless much concerned with the humane treatment of experimental animals. To begin his search for a more suitable anesthetic for his surgical procedures, he consulted his colleague, Hanriot, director of the chemistry laboratory that was close by his own. Richet suggested to Hanriot that he make a combination of chloral hydrate with lactic acid. The idea seemed worth testing because lactic acid was known to accumulate in the body in association with muscular fatigue which in turn was often followed by sleep. Unfortunately, the mixture proved to be a powerful convulsant. Later Hanriot found that combining chloral hydrate with glucose yielded a plain white powder, sparingly soluble in warm water, that seemed ideal for an anesthetic; it suppressed or abolished pain and inhibited muscular activity without lowering blood pressure or impairing other vital functions.[R 346] As Richet stated, "it put the cerebral hemispheres to sleep but excited the medulla."[R 736] In fact neuromuscular reflexes and autonomic responses were enhanced by chloralose, as they named it. The accentuation of reflex functions proved advantageous in some neurophysiological studies so that, despite its poor solubility, chloralose is still widely used by neuroscientists today.

Soon after Richet's discovery, chloralose had also found favor as a painkiller and hypnotic for patients. For a time it was relied upon by some of the leading French internists, including Louis Joseph Landouzy and Pierre Marie (1853-1940). Richet tells of one of Landouzy's patients, the wife of a prominent politician. Suffering severely from insomnia and wishing to commit suicide, she consumed a very large dose (four grams) of chloralose. Although she slept for forty-eight hours she had no ill effects, cardiovascular or otherwise. Ultimately, despite its relative safety and effectiveness, chloralose was abandoned by most clinicians because of its tendency to accentuate autonomic reflexes, thereby raising blood pressure or altering heart rate. It continued to be used in surgical shock, however, where the need was to sustain or even elevate blood pressure. Therefore, during World War I Richet took chloralose to the front by ambulance for use in surgical procedures on soldiers whose degree of blood loss had rendered too hazardous the use of ether or chloroform as an anesthetic.

Ironically, despite Richet's introduction of a humane anesthetic for animals and, although he was recognized by his colleagues as one who cared for the comfort and welfare of his animals, he continued to be attacked by antivivisectionists and was often harassed by the press for his use of animals in research. In fact, he may have had doubts and inner conflicts about the propriety of vivisection. His book of poetry, *Pour les Grands et le Petits* contains a poem that suggests an ambivalence about the use of animals in experimentation. While the poem was apparently written to express Richet's democratic and pacifistic convictions, it recounts the efforts of a medical scientist to persuade an unwilling rabbit to submit to vivisection. The scientist argues that a discovery could bring glory to both him and the rabbit. Since the rabbit would not cooperate, however, the experimenter was forced to let him go to have time to repent his failure to realize his opportunity for glory, and ultimately be reduced to the lowly destiny of eating cabbage leaves.

LE LAPIN ET LE SAVANT

Jeannot lapin, l'infortuné
Au logis d'un savant fut amené.
Ces savants ont une âme dure,
Ils se plaisent dans la torture.
De maint animal innocent,
Espérant arracher à la mère nature
Quelques secrets au prix de sang.
Donc, notre savant détestable
Mit Jeannot lapin sur la table;
Mais Jeannot lapin resistait
Secouant sa tête meurtrie
En des soubessants de furie
Comme un démon il s'agitait.
"Indocile animal, stupide créature,"
Dit le professeur irrité,
"Pour une méchante piqure
C'est bien du bruit, en vérité!
Tu fais preuve à mes yeux d'une ignorance extrême;
Car, si je m'occupais de toi,
C'etait pour éclaircir un étonnant problème;
C'etait pour resoudre une loi
Qui, si tu comprenais, t'éblouirait toi-même.

Je sais que ce raisonnement
Dépasse de beaucoup ton humble sapience;
Mais laisse-moi tranquillement
Poursuivre mon expérience.
Je vais près de ton coeur, enfoncer mes ciseaux,—
La tentative est delicate—
J'enlève ces deux petits os,
Et c'est fini, foi d'Hippocrate.
Quand le succès n'est pas douteux
Souffrir un peu, c'est peu de chose;
Songe que tu soutiens une sublime cause,
Et que notre gloire à tous deux
Sur ton seul courage repose.
N'es tu pas mieux pourvu que tes aieux obscurs?
Pour quelques moments un peu durs,
Pauvres inconnus que nous sommes,
On nous célèbrera dans les âges futurs
Comme les bienfaiteurs des lapins et des hommes.
A ce discours rempli d'appât,
Le lapin ne repondit pas.
Il se démena de plus belle,
Si bien que, le trouvant à ses projets rebelle,
L'opérateur dut le laisser partir.
Hélas! Jeannot lapin eut à s'en repentir;
Car il vécut longtemps, mais il vécut sans gloire
Un chou fut tout son histoire.
Petit peuple menu fretin,
C'est pour vous que j'ai fait ce conte.
Suivez l'exemple du lapin,
Vous y trouverez votre compte.
N' écoutez pas les potentats,
Puissant conducteurs des états,
Qui vous rebattent les oreilles
De la gloire et de ses merveilles,
Faisant luire à vos yeux, pour la postérité
L'éspoir d'un vain éclat chèrement mérité.
. . . .
Gens de peu, gens de rien, ne soyez pas si bêtes!
Laissez les empéreurs faire seuls leurs conquètes,
Et sachez, restant sourds aux clairons des tyrans,
Que le sang des petits fait la gloire des grands.

THE RABBIT AND THE SCIENTIST

Unfortunate Johnny Rabbit
Brought into the laboratory
Where hard hearted scientists
Enjoy the act of torture,
Hoping to extract from mother nature
Her secrets in exchange for Johnny's blood.
The scientist puts Johnny on the table
But Johnny struggles to get free.
He twists and turns his body to escape.
"Indocile animal, stupid creature,"
The angry scientist complained.
A simple needle prick
Brings out in you an unbecoming fury
Which proves to me your utter ignorance.
Since I concern myself with you
It is to clarify a stunning truth,
Establish an enduring law
Which, you see, would make you great.
I know this explanation far
Exceeds the range of your poor brain
But let me quietly
Pursue my master plan
To plunge these scissors near your heart,
A delicate maneuver,
To cut away two little bones
And that is all. It's finished then.
When there's no doubt of outcome
A bit of pain's a small price to pay.
Your contribution to the cause
Brings glory to us both.
From your courage you'd surpass
Your mediocre friends in rabbit land.
For only moments of enduring pain
We poor unknowns become at once
Renowned and esteemed in future years
As benefactors both of men and rabbits.
To this harangue designed to charm
Young Johnny offered no reply.
Instead he struggled all the more
So all his tormentor could do
Was to let him go and lose his chance for fame.
Alas he dispatched the rabbit to repent.
Although he lived, instead of glory

A cabbage leaf became his prize.
Youngsters who are offered trash
For you I've made this tale.
Follow the path of the rabbit
To find your destiny.
Ignore the greedy potentates,
Ambitious crafty heads of state
Who fill your ears with mighty tales
Of conquest and of glory
To coax your eyes to shine with hope
For future vain and costly benefit.
. . . .
Poor and ordinary folks be not so foolish
Let the emperors seek their own triumphs.
Be deaf to the bugle sounds of tyrants
Lest the blood of the people buy glory for their rulers.

Passive Immunization (Serotherapy)

In 1887, the year of his appointment as professor, while exploring the possibility of an infectious origin of cancer, Richet injected under the skin of a dog an extract isolated from a subcutaneous tumor in another dog. The tumor had apparently been infected by a staphylococcus. When only an abscess resulted, he tried inoculating rabbits with the organism. This time the result was fatal staphylococcal septicemia. Recalling a report attributed to Chauveau that sheep, having been exposed to anthrax, were immune to the disease, Richet and his colleague, Héricourt, successfully protected rabbits against the staphylococcus infection by injecting them intraperitoneally with blood from the dog from which the staphylococcus had been isolated. Their paper reporting this important discovery was rejected for publication in the *Archives de Médecine Expérimentale* by its editor, Isidore Straus (1845–1896). Richet was furious, reacting as if Straus were guilty of lèse majesté. "Straus was jealous," wrote Richet, " . . . peevish, dissatisfied with everything." I had never before had one of my papers rejected by a publisher," he wrote. The findings were later presented to the Académie des Sciences 5 November 1888 and published in the *Comptes Rendus de l'Académie des Sciences*.[R230] "The report was received with indifference, even hostility" wrote Richet, "only my excellent friend Adolph Pinard understood the significance of the work" (Unp).

Conceptions of disease and immunity at that time were guided by the work of Louis Pasteur whose focus was on external agents (bacteria). An animal was thought to enjoy immunity if its tissues did not provide a suitable medium for the replication of microbes. René Jules DuBos (1901-1982) a world renowned microbiologist stated Pasteur's view of acquired immunity as follows: "Microbial agents of disease refuse to grow in a body which they have previously invaded: this body has been depleted by the first invasion of some factor essential for growth." Later Pasteur developed an alternative hypothesis that somehow bacterial growth, adds new substances to the tissues of the host that inhibit its own further replication. Richet, in contrast, proposed that the presumed immunizing substance was produced, not by the bacteria, but by the host itself. Thus the function of serotherapy was to transfer an immunizing substance produced by an animal that had recovered from an infection to another animal, thereby rendering it immune to the infective agent. It appears that most of the scientific establishment failed to recognize the conceptual contribution in Richet's demonstration of passive immunity.

Unfortunately, instead of adhering to the commitment to physiology that he expressed in his first lecture and trying to discover the underlying mechanisms responsible for passive immunity, Richet, with his colleague, Héricourt began a lengthy and ultimately futile foray into medical therapeutics. They decided to test the possibility of a practical application of serotherapy against a widely prevalent and potentially fatal disease. They considered several, including diphtheria, but selected tuberculosis because it was the most prevalent disease in France and had the greatest social impact throughout Europe at that time. They began an intense but disappointing ten-year effort to develop a serum, first against tuberculosis and then against cancer. So many animals were required for the work that Richet was forced to rent a place at Joinville Le Pont to house them. In his laboratory there was room for only six or eight dogs. Although results continued to be unpromising, a human trial was undertaken 6 December 1890 on a tuberculous patient on Verneuil's service at Hôtel Dieu. He and Héricourt injected the patient with a serum prepared from his tuberculous dogs. There is no record of the outcome in this patient, but Richet's experiments with tuberculous dogs were disappointing. None were cured and Richet eventually abandoned the effort.

Meanwhile, Emil von Behring (1854-1917), an assistant to Robert Koch (1843-1910), had achieved an immune serum that protected people against diphtheria and tetanus. His work had been stimulated by that of Pierre Paul Emile Roux (1853–1933) who in 1888 with Alexandre Emile Jean Yersin (1863–1943) discovered that the diphtheria bacillus produces a toxin (Roux & Yersin). Although Roux modestly demurred, the French press credited him as the father of serotherapy much to the disgust of Charles Richet.

Conflict over Credit for Priority

Von Behring's publication, co-authored with Shibasaburo Kitasato (1852–1931) appeared in the *Deutsche Medizinische Wochenschrift* (von Behring 1890). It failed to acknowledge the work of Héricourt and Richet published two years earlier. Indeed, Von Behring later wrote that Richet's work was "speculation on natural philosophy" (von Behring 1890). For the rest of his life Richet remained bitter about von Behring's failure to acknowledge his priority. Von Behring, for his part, was scornful of the worldwide acclaim he received: "Tous les prix qu'on me décerne, je m'en moque. Je ne tiens qu'a la somme d'argent qu'ils représentment."[9]

Although in his *Leçon Inaugurale* Richet had declared that the experimental laboratory was the source of sound clinical knowledge, he opted to defer testing his brilliant intuition that immunity is produced by the response of an invaded body rather than being due to the direct action of an invading organism as Pasteur had proposed. He thus abandoned any attempt to unravel the mechanisms of immunity by experimentation in favor of prompt therapeutic application which consumed a great deal of his time and energy without significant yield.

Serotherapy for Cancer

Richet seized an opportunity to test the possibility of immunization against cancer offered in 1894 by the affliction of his sister-in-law's sixteen-year-old daughter, Amélie Vian, with an abdominal cancer. He and Héricourt began experimental treatments on cancerous humans using serum from a dog that had been injected with an extract of a human tumor, an osteosarcoma obtained from the surgeon, Jean Jacques Reclus (1847–1914). Reclus and another surgeon Louis Felix Terrier (1837–1914) each treated a patient with repeated subcutaneous injections of the serum. In the patient of Reclus, suffering from cancer of the stomach, the treatment seemed to work wonderfully well, "Marvelous" Richet recalled, "I was dazzled, more so than ever before. Never have I had comparable emotions. The pain ceased, the tumor diminished and began to wither." (Unp) At that point the patient left the hospital and was not seen again. Terrier's patient, who was thought to have a sarcoma of the arm, also improved without operation but on later biopsy the tumor turned out to be a benign fibroma. Treatments continued and, according to Richet, some of the patients seemed to improve remarkably. He wrote, "Their appetite and strength returned—but this improvement did not last." After two or three months there was less and less improvement and more urticaria and joint pains.[10] Other patients reacted similarly. Convinced that the early favorable results had not been due to chance, Richet published his findings[R][396] and soon was deluged with requests for the serum by pitiful victims and families of victims of cancer. Although there was an initial remission in many, in none was it possible to prevent a fatal outcome so the treatments were stopped.

Richet, convinced that the principle of immunotherapy for cancer was valid and would ultimately yield a useful treatment, wrote in his *Mémoires* "It is also likely that anti-cancer serotherapy, which since 1895 has given us the most encouraging results, has not said the last word, and that the investigations undertaken on every side with so much ardor to illuminate the aetiology of the disease will find their application on the preparation of curative serum." Even in his article on immunity in the *Dictionnaire de Physiologie*. Charles Richet devoted nearly two pages to the consideration of the future possibilities of immunization against cancer. He concluded, "immunity against cancer, natural or acquired, has been thus far barely approached. But well established facts, though few in number, are sufficient for us to hope for a solution in the future."

It is typical of his prescience that, nearly a hundred years after Richet's abortive attempt at an immunologic treatment for cancer, patients today are being treated immunologically with injections of antibodies prepared by the methods of modern molecular biology against the specific cells of the invading cancer (Wright 1984; Baldwin & Byers 1986). Frank H. DeLand in his 1989 essay on *A perspective of monoclonal antibodies: past, present & future* wrote, "The methods of Héricourt and Richet were quite similar to those first used in the middle of this century, albeit less sophisticated" (DeLand 1989).

Zomotherapy

Still not moved to return to the laboratory and explore further a well-documented effect that he had discovered, Richet, as it were, jumped from the frying pan into the fire to further pursue uncontrolled therapeutics. As he recounted in his *Mémoires*, "One day when we still had one inoculated dog (the others having died of TB) the idea came to me to feed him raw meat because of a vague notion that by metabolizing meat alone, uric acid would be produced in greater quantity. Moreover, TB is rare among people with gout—more or less mediocre and uncertain ideas." The dog did very well and seemingly recovered. Richet then confirmed the experiment with several other dogs that he inoculated with tuberculosis. He further found that cooked meat did not have the same salutary effect as the raw product. Initial results of repeated experiments with controls seemed immensely encouraging. Some of the dogs fed raw meat recovered completely and survived for many years. Richet found a rationale for his therapy in that clinicians had used raw meat to treat the diarrhea of TB. After the diarrhea subsided their patients were customarily returned to a normal diet. The enthusiastic Richet, with his colleague Héricourt, began to treat tuberculous patients with raw meat. As some of them seemed to improve, the work aroused a good deal of interest throughout Paris.

One day, after a lecture on the new therapy at the Sorbonne, Richet was approached by a city official named Ambroise Rendu who told him of a bequest of 1,500,000 francs that had been made to Paris by two ladies, Mesdames Jouye and Tanies, for medical facilities for the poor. Rendu offered to establish a hospital facility in the relatively impoverished twentieth arrondissement for the treatment of tuberculosis with raw meat juice. Richet readily agreed and the project was activated with Héricourt serving as physician in charge. Although initial results seemed excellent, there was no arrangement to follow up the patients after discharge. Other physicians, who tried the treatment, found it less effective. Nevertheless, Richet continued to be proud of his achievement and considered what he had begun to call zomotherapy (from *zomos*, Greek for bouillon or meat juice), to have been one of his major contributions. He explained the failure of the general medical profession to confirm his findings as due to the fact that they did not use enough meat juice. Also he added that "doctors always resist new things" (Unp).

Just prior to World War I Richet had arranged with two chemists named Grigaut and Guilbaud for the production in Argentina of freeze-dried beef juice named Zomine. He further arranged for his son Albert to manage the factory. Albert had been an aeronautic engineer and wanted a change of career. The plan was interrupted by the war in which Albert served as a fighter pilot and was killed. After the war Richet was able to make other arrangements for production with the help of an industrialist from Le Havre named Latham. Richet continued to pursue the therapeutic possibilities of zomotherapy (the feeding of raw beef juice) for several years without developing a strategy to test the validity of his optimistic assessments of the treatment, or to explore the mechanisms of its action. The results of his beef juice treatment, which Richet interpreted as highly successful, are described in his monograph *La Nouvelle Zomothérapie*.[R 644]

Contrasting with this remarkably uncritical and pedestrian therapeutic venture that could hardly be dignified as research, was an imaginative and well controlled inquiry into the changing characteristics of microbes mentioned in chapter 4.

Experiments with Microbes and Metals

While working in the laboratory of Berthelot in 1877, Richet had become interested in the chemical and microbiological aspects of the fermentation of milk, a subject that had been richly explored by his scientific idol, Pasteur. In his *Souvenirs d'un Physiologiste*,[R 736] Richet described in detail the meticulous precautions required in order to properly observe and modify the process of fermentation. Milk was a convenient vehicle because, as Richet showed, fermentation of milk in the presence of oxygen produces butyric acid, while anaerobic fermentation (lacking oxygen) produces lactic acid. Thus fermentation could be quantified by measuring the amount of lactic or butyric acid produced. As Richet recorded in his *Mémoires*, "for fifty years I pursued the study of the fermentation of milk which gave me many remarkable results." In the series of experiments described in chapter 4, Richet found that the slowly progressive exposure of a culture of lactobacilli in milk to metallic salts enabled the organisms, through successive generations, to acquire immunity to what had previously been a fatal dose of the metallic salt.[R 421; 541; 597; 618; 629; 630]

What Richet and his collaborators had observed and reported was the now familiar phenomenon of resistance to antimicrobial agents. Only years later, with the widespread use of antibiotics in medicine and animal husbandry, which has led to increased growth and survival of drug-resistant mutant forms, was the phenomenon of antibiotic resistance generally recognized and ultimately understood.

Paul Ehrlich (1854–1915) in 1907 had also observed such resistance in cultures of deadly trypanosome parasites grown in the presence of a chemical that was initially highly effective against the disease that they caused. Eventually, however, the organisms in culture developed resistance to the previously effective chemical (Ehrlich 1907). In 1945, when penicillin came into general use, mutant strains of bacteria emerged that were not only resistant to the drug but eventually became dependent on penicillin for survival (Davis 1967). Later, the work of Jacques Lucien Monod (1910–1976), André Michael Lwoff (1902–) and François Jacob (1920–) explained the phenomenon of resistance as due to enzymatic induction of a penicillin antagonist through genetic mutation. For this and related discoveries, which did much to launch the science of molecular biology, they shared the Nobel Prize in physiology and medicine in 1965.

Unfortunately neither Ehrlich nor Richet are usually credited with the discovery of the phenomenon of resistance developing in successive generations of microbes exposed to a toxic agent. Unfamiliar at that time with genetic mutations, Richet had failed to isolate a single colony (of mutated bacteria) and propagate it as a pure culture of metal resistant organisms. Moreover, he had interpreted his important discovery as supporting the then widely accepted theory of inherited transmission of acquired characteristics.[R614] Propounded in the early nineteenth-century, the theory had later become associated with Lamarck. It was finally rejected to be superseded by the new knowledge of mutant selection in genetics. Recently, however, interest in the possibility of inheriting acquired adaptations has been revived (Aufderheide 1980).[11]

Richet's studies of metallic poisons also led him to another discovery with broad biological significance. He observed that among salts of metals that are found in the same column of the periodic table[12] the rarer ones in nature, cesium, as compared to potassium, for example, strontium to calcium and cadmium to zinc, were relatively more toxic than their more abundant partners that play an essential role in the bodily economy of man and other animals.[93; 356] Richet inferred that the requirement for such metals had evolved during gradual evolutionary adaptation to their ubiquity in the environment. As he put it, "Living beings from their origin have had to adapt to chemical environments as a result they have become accustomed to this or that chemical substance. The earth and the sea are rich in the salts of potassium and sodium. Hence these salts would naturally be less toxic."

A less felicitous study with bacteria involved an attempt to sterilize a broth culture by filtering it through a porous substance. After two years without success, Richet learned that Charles Edouard Chamberland (1851–1908) had previously succeeded in doing so.[R 120] A different sort of disappointment greeted a set of successful experiments Richet carried out after World War I with his daughter Adèle Le Ber. They grew various plants including wheat, beans, and onions in sterilized earth and found that growth was greatly enhanced. Afterwards they learned that an English botanical chemist, John Edward Russell (1872–1917) had already made that discovery.[R 631]

Gliding and Powered Flight

Richet had acquired an interest in aeronautics from Marey, who, with the aid of his *fusil photographique*, already described, had discovered some of the laws of aerodynamics from his study of birds in flight. In 1888 one of Marey's laboratory associates, a highly skilled engineer named Victor Tatin, hoping to enable humans to fly, constructed a flying machine with flapping wings powered by a small steam engine. The internal combustion engine had not as yet been perfected. Tatin's unmanned machine, tested in the courtyard of the Collège de France, could fly only twenty or thirty meters, after which it fell to the ground and broke up.

Confident that powered flight was possible, Marey suggested to Richet that he work with Tatin on the interesting problem of aviation. Richet's acquaintance with the subject was confined to a lively fascination with the books of Jules Verne and an experience in a glider with a famous glider pilot named Godart. On that occasion, no sooner were they in the air then Richet realized that Godart was drunk. (Unp) Fortunately they were able to land without incident. Marey's suggestion stimulated

Richet's imagination. He thereupon eagerly added another field of endeavor to his already multiple activities.

In 1888, soon after beginning to work with Tatin, Richet suggested that they abandon the flapping wing design in favor of a fixed single-winged arrangement similar to that of a glider or of an albatross maneuvering among air currents.[13] Their new plane was propelled by an air screw powered by a small steam engine. Richet's single-wing idea anticipated the fuselage design of the monoplane, without which the era of modern high speed, long flight aviation would not have been possible. Later, a monoplane designed by Duperdussin won the Gordon Bennett cup in 1913 but the single-wing design met general acceptance only after World War I.

The trials of Richet's new single-wing plane were carried out near Le Havre at Cap La Hève on the channel coast, and at Carqueiranne in Provence. The unmanned machine succeeded in flying 875 meters in a straight line after being launched from a steep slope on the Normandy Cliffs. The experimenters made fewer trials than they should have, because, as Richet put it, "we had the absurd idea that we could fly only when there was no wind and this was a rare circumstance on the seashore." After their partial success, however, working in a hangar at Carqueiranne they began to construct a machine powered by an internal combustion engine capable of carrying two passengers. By now (1898) such engines had reached a sufficient stage of development to be light enough to be airborne. Richet, eager to be the first to fly, but mindful of the possibility of an unwanted dip in the ocean, had to learn to swim at the age of forty-eight.

Later the two hopeful aviators were joined by the two sons of Antoine Breguet, Richet's close friend who had worked with him in the study of summation of visual stimuli and as co-editor of *La Revue Scientifique*, but who died in 1882 at age thirty-one.[14]

Richet had promised Antoine before he died that he would look after his two sons. Both boys, Louis now eighteen and Jacques now seventeen, were vigorous, enthusiastic youngsters. The aircraft project seemed ideal to keep them occupied and interested.

For the next six years, Richet, Tatin, and the boys worked furiously on the project, frequently modifying and perfecting the design of the aircraft. By 1904 they were nearly ready for an attempt at manned flight, but their efforts were eclipsed when Orville and Wilbur Wright succeeded in flying their plane a distance of a few kilometers. Not long afterward Victor Tatin died of cancer of the tongue. "Tatin was unable to participate in the triumph of aviation," wrote Richet, "how painful it is to think that he was never accorded his proper credit." Louis Breguet, however, went on to a distinguished career in the manufacture of aircraft. In 1907, with his brother Jacques, he founded France's first, and for many years largest, aircraft company, Breguet Aviation, originally called Ateliers Breguet-Richet. With Richet the two brothers designed a helicopter which they called a gyroplane. Within the first year their creation, carrying engine and pilot, rose 60 centimeters from the ground. Two years later in 1909 the plane made its first real solo flight with Louis as pilot. Soon thereafter, when Richet's interests had shifted to other concerns, the company's name was changed to Société Anonyme des Ateliers d'Aviation Louis Breguet. Jacques by now was in poor health, although he did not die until 1939.

Strangely, and despite the obvious success of the monoplane in the Gordon Bennett Air Show, Breguet did not early adopt Richet's forward-looking monoplane design for commercial aircraft manufacture. Nevertheless, the biplanes of Breguet must have contributed importantly to the Allied success in World War I. Richet, in his *Souvenirs d'un Physiologiste* wrote, "I can justifiably say (with some pride) that because of me Louis Breguet was able to become the biggest manufacturer of flying machines in the world.[R 736] For a few years Richet continued his relationship with the Breguets, providing financial backing as well as helping design the early helicopter.

In an address to his fellow physiologists in Vienna in 1910, Richet, deploring his government's inadequate support of science, cited aviation, made possible by the research of the Wright Brothers,[R 615] to illustrate the social benefits of research and experimentation. He could not resist, however, giving primary credit to a Frenchman, his old chief Marey, for his fundamental contributions to aerodynamics and his "sagacity in predicting the triumph of the airman." Neither could he resist claiming credit for himself as well. "With my ingenious friend, Tatin, in 1892 we constructed and launched the first airplane." Paradoxically, in his later years, when enthusiasts began to explore the possibilities of flight in space, Richet was both doubtful and scornful.[R 686] It has often been said that great strides in any field of science may delay or inhibit the next important development. The long halt in developments in medical teaching that followed the signal contributions of Claudius Galen (129-200) is a classical case in point. Thus, the final realization of man's dream to fly may have contributed to restraining the usually bold foresight of Richet. Concerning the future possibility of flight in space he wrote with Latin emphasis: "Et nati natorum et qui nascentur ab illis" Never, never will we be able to leave our earth.[R 607] He added, "Ingenious dreamers have supposed that certain powerful machines, huge projectiles containing men, could be flown into space beyond the limits of gravity to reach the moon or one of the planets of the solar system. Let us resign ourselves. The rock does not expect to walk on the waves. The tree in the forest does not lament because it cannot gambol across the fields with the leaves and the seed pods, so man should not be more ambitious because, like the rock on the mountain and the tree in the forest, he is also tightly adherent to the earth."[R 686]

A Private Island in the Mediterranean

After his father's death Richet, seeking solitude and quiet for his writing found managing the large château at Carqueiranne somewhat burdensome. It no longer afforded him the haven for escape from the distractions of Paris and the opportunity to read, write, fish, and think without interruption. One source of disturbance was the farm manager, Latty, who often took over the château when there were no family members present. He gave large dinners and parties for his friends in the neighborhood, altered the landscape by cutting down trees, and generally behaved without restraint. Latty's ne'er-do-well son contracted syphilis and infected a young girl from a neighborhood family. Richet was fond of the girl and he became embittered when she subsequently died of syphilitic meningitis. In his *Mémoires* he recalled his need for a more secluded environment where he could write, relax and enjoy the company of a few choice guests.

From a friend, Louis Gaidan, Richet learned of a small island that was for sale, the Île Ribaud. It lay just off the Mediterranean coast near Giens, east of Toulon. There were no buildings on it except for a lighthouse and an abandoned fort that had been active during the Napoleonic wars. The price was 16,000 francs. His wife opposed the purchase but agreed to their assuming part ownership, sharing the cost with his old friends Louis

Gaidan, Gaston Fournier, brother of Paul, and Richet's cousin Philippe
Renouard. The purchase was concluded June 12, 1897.

Île Ribaud is one of the Îles d'Hyères, a group of once nearly deserted
island jewels covered with unusually rare, interesting and fragrant veg-
etation. They have been dear to many distinguished Frenchmen. François
Rabelais (1494–1553) had claimed to be the *calloier* of the Îles
d'Hyères.[15] When, in his latter years Richet was interviewed by Albert
Jay Nock, author of *A Journey into Rabelais's France*, Richet remarked
that "the French, especially the Parisians, do not like to cross the water
and, even though the crossing to the islands is so short, they balk at it."
"Hence," he said, "visitors rarely approach these shores; but I must admit
that does not distress me. My sentiment is divided. On the one hand, I
could wish these marvelous islands to become well known, much fre-
quented, highly celebrated. On the other hand, I dread the swarming-in
of a mediocre type of visitor, mere wanderers in quest of emotional
stirrings, tourists hard-bound in vulgarity and snobbery, to dishonor this
abode of peace and beauty." When asked why he spent much of his time
there Richet replied,

> By living in the world of men, one ends perforce by losing one's identity; all one's
> differentiating originality disappears. One ceases to think for oneself for the sake of
> thinking like others; which is equivalent to no longer thinking at all. One gasps for
> breath in an unwholesome and profitless palpitation, like the squirrel driving the wheel
> of his cage around and around to no purpose; and in spite of all the silly responsibilities
> that are piled on us, all the words we speak and all the mechanical measures that we
> multiply, one has only the illusion of activity.

> But here, looking out upon an ever-changing sea, under a sun that is always kindly,
> among trees that are always green, one's true activity, that is to say the activity of the
> spirit, has a free rein. Here one indulges in activity of an indisputably higher order
> than the activity of doing; it is the activity of dreaming. For poets, artists, scholars,
> nothing else is worth as much as a few weeks of isolation and reflection in these dear
> islands. One sloughs off one's grubby vanities and harassing cares; one becomes once
> more a personality; one strengthens one's inner life, which is the only true life one
> has. (Nock 1934)

Richet kept motor boats and sailboats on hand for visits to mainland
ports, racing and fishing. One was named for his wife Amélie. Others
were named Circé, Feu Follet, and Lutétia. The lighthouse tender, who
remained on the island throughout the year, served as caretaker. Richet
tried to establish colonies of several types of animals on the island

including kangaroos. The kangaroos reproduced only once and within the next year they all died.

By the early 1900s Richet had acquired Fournier's share in the island and after World War II his children and the Renouards bought Gaidan's interest; thereby the Richets retained a two-thirds share of the property with the Renouards holding the other one-third. Charles built a family house and an adjoining house for servants. On a high knoll about 200 yards from the houses he built a two- story tower with an open terrace on top from which he could scan the whole island, the shore and the sea. The bedroom beneath was his own while the one at ground level was for servants and visitors. For the subsequent years of Richet's professorship and beyond, Île Ribaud played an important part in his life. Distinguished visitors were entertained, plans were concocted and deals agreed upon on his lovely wild island.

A Family Disaster

Richet and his sister, who had become major shareholders in the *Revue des Deux Mondes*, participated with her husband, Charles Buloz, the editor, in directing its literary content. Richet liked his brother-in-law. As he put it, "I was in perfect harmony with him. I knew he was very shallow, incapable of serious discussion, but he was sociable and pleasant, a good fellow. Nevertheless I had a vague, uneasy feeling that something was wrong." It was; Richet learned later that Buloz had squandered the journal's funds. To protect his sister, Richet demanded and obtained Buloz' power of attorney, paid the bills from his own funds and in the course of investigation discovered that the journal's account books had been falsified. There was soon a call for a court hearing. To avoid that and the possible imprisonment of Buloz, Richet had to obtain 700,000 francs, a very large sum at that time, within a period of 24 hours. Doing so required the liquidation of some of Louise's as well as his own assets. The financial burden was extremely heavy for Charles and Louise. They had to sell Epinay and mortgage the house at 15 rue de l'Université. Their stock in *Revue des Deux Mondes* was now worth very little. Louise promptly separated from her husband Buloz who died of cancer of the tongue four years later. She eventually remarried a close friend, Louis Joseph Landouzy, a prominent internist who had recently been widowed. Buloz' assistant, Ferdinand Brunetière, who had been virtually in charge for the preceding ten years during Buloz' adventures, succeeded to the post of editor of the *Revue*. Richet was not happy with his leadership because he sensed that Brunetière "in an insidious way, had developed into a fierce clericalist—he who had been a free thinker and reasonably revolutionary." The character of the journal changed and income decreased.

Richet was always at his best in crisis. When Buloz disclosed his misappropriation of the journal's funds Richet quickly took charge and, despite the later dispiriting revelation of fraud, he displayed fortitude, valor, and even magnanimity. Although he was faced with a serious threat to his family and good name he was able to maintain a remarkable self-possession throughout. His grandson, Gabriel, considered such behavior characteristic of his grandfather. "Whatever event affected his family, France or the world," he said, "Charles Richet felt a responsibility to be involved. Involvement runs in our family."

In 1917, twenty-four years after the devastating Buloz affair both Landouzy and Louise died. Thereafter, in summing up Buloz' behavior, Richet commented, "Although he did a great deal of harm to my sister he was not a bad man. He was mainly stupid, unalterably stupid. He spent money here and there without being concerned about the time when nothing would be left. Since he had absolutely no notion of morality he did not hesitate to take money wherever he found it with no thought of the future and without asking himself whether it was right or wrong to do so." In later years Richet wrote warmly of Buloz: "In so far as possible, my dear children, remember him kindly despite his faults, his misdeeds and his near crimes that might cast a dark shadow on his reputation." (Unp)

Richet's failure to gain insight into the character of his brother-in-law, Charles Buloz, even after years of knowing him and working closely with him on the *Revue des Deux Mondes*, is perhaps indicative of his emotional aloofness from most people, demanding from them only charm and good manners. The Richet-Buloz relationship had not been close but was rather one of "class solidarity." Buloz betrayed his class and thus, in Richet's view, he fell into obscurity.

A Publishing Venture

His grandfather's love of books and his own made it seem appropriate for Richet to try to interest his much loved cousin, Philippe Renouard, in the publishing business. As he put it, "the great grandsons of Antoine Auguste Renouard were destined at birth to be bibliophiles, bibliographers, and publishers." They began a collection of sixteenth-century French works, looking especially for books published by their great grandfather from 1796–1825. A catalogue of their books was published at a printing press on the Boulevard St. Germain in the same building where Richet's *Revue Scientifique* was produced. From a chance meeting with an Englishman Richet learned of a newly developed composing machine, the linotype. With his usual partiality toward innovation, Richet bought it for Philippe who then hired a printer and moved to a new site on rue Pont de Lodi near the home of Richet's friend Henri Ferrari. Later Richet arranged a merger with another publisher named Chamerot. The new enterprise, located at 15 rue des Saints Pères, was called "L'imprimerie Chamerot-Renouard." A few years later Chamerot retired, leaving the business to Philippe. Richet's twenty-year-old son, Jacques was then brought into the firm. The books were of high quality, perhaps too high for the clientele and ultimately the business failed.

Historical Interests

Richet had a deep interest in history but deplored the way most historians built the continuity of their work around military conquests instead of tracing the intellectual, civil, and social progress of mankind. He objected especially to the proclivity of historians to glorify and romanticize military leaders. Toward Napoleon's exploits, for example, Richet held a view that most of his French compatriots could not have shared. "Posterity has been unjust (to Napoleon)," he wrote, "by excessive leniency." He further commented, "this emperor, who crushed all liberty under his heel, this merciless soldier, this implacable despot, has been transformed into a fatherly, good natured sovereign wearing a grey frock coat and a little hat, full of care for the meek and lowly and delivering the poor from their servitude to the church. To the impartial view, Napoleon was the most evil of mortals. Through him the human race has been debased" (Unp.).

Richet's fascination with history was reflected in the way he began many of his lectures and publications by laying a fairly lengthy historical background. Early in his career he had become interested in the history of medicine and science. He wrote a discourse on Michael Servetus

$(1511-1553)^{R\,677}$ and dozens of forewords for books by colleagues, and arranged for the reprinting of classical works by French medical scientists including Marie François Xavier Bichat (1771-1802), Lavoisier and other distinguished Europeans, among them Lazzaro Spallanzani and John Hunter (1728-1793).

In 1912 Richet wrote a book, *Abrégé d'histoire générale*, a short history of civilization, conceived, as he put it, "in the spirit of pacifism."[R 533] Writing in a popular, almost breezy style, Richet described people of Western civilizations, their customs and beliefs and the events they created. His text began in prehistory and extended through what he called the despotic eras in Egypt, the Near Eastern empires, Greece, Rome, and Christendom for the years 312 to 1450. He traced developments in science from 1789 to 1914, giving French science the most attention, but also acknowledging the work of prominent foreigners, including Galileo Galilei (1564-1642), Bacon, Harvey, Leibniz, Sir Isaac Newton (1643-1727), and Christiaan Huygens (1629-1695). Andrew Carnegie, who learned about the book during its preparation, offered to have it translated into several languages. Hachette, publisher of the French edition, delivered the proofs to Richet on 20 July 1914, but because Richet was fully occupied with his wartime commitments, the French edition did not appear until 1919. A German translation was published in 1917, however, thanks to Richet's having given a copy of his manuscript to his friend, Dr. Rudolph Berger. Later Carnegie arranged for translations into other languages.

Bibliographical Activities

Richet was concerned about keeping track of the burgeoning literature in physiology and medicine. He, therefore, in 1894 launched a new publication, *Bibliographica Physiologica*, adapting the decimal system which had been introduced by Melvil Dewey (1851-1931) shortly before.[R377] His first problem was to decide what to include. It was especially difficult to select from the massive literature of medicine and surgery those contributions most relevant to physiology. For his first volume Richet finally settled on 3200 papers and books published in 1893-1894.

Richet himself had provided most of the money for the enterprise although Henri de Rothschild contributed 6,000 francs in exchange for sixty subscriptions. He then sold the subscriptions at a reduced rate much to Richet's distress. In the end there were less than 200 subscriptions sold including Rothschild's sixty. Richet was, therefore, forced to abandon the project after publishing only two issues. The idea was taken up by the Royal Society of London under the imprimatur of the International Association of Academies. They produced what Richet considered an elegant publication but, since they used a decimal system for cataloging other than Dewey's, Richet turned instead to John Shaw Billings' Index Catalogue published by the U.S. Surgeon General in Washington. Billings had sent a yearly subscription to Richet as a gift. At that time the only other French subscriber to the Index Catalogue was Jacques Raphael (1840-1919) at Lyon.

Next Richet, with a small coterie of bright and eager collaborators, undertook the task of editing a compendium of all extant knowledge of physiology. He recruited an international panel of contributors in addition to his laboratory associates. Each was to provide a richly annotated bibliography on one or more topics to be arranged alphabetically in the book. Again Richet was faced with the problem of which topics to cover and which to omit. Histology was omitted because, as Richet expressed it, "Histology seemed to me fairly useless to physiology." The first volume of the work, *Dictionnaire de Physiologie*, was published in 1895.[R 391] The first topic "Abasia-Astasia" cited only two references, Blocq's original description of the condition in 1888 and Charcot's textbook based on his experience at Salpêtière.

The series of volumes, one appearing each year, was interrupted by World War I, the last entry in the 1914 edition being "Luminescence." After the war one additional volume was produced in 1923, extending the alphabet only through "Moelle Epinière" (spinal cord). The article was written by George Charles Guillain (1876-1961). Up to that point the *Dictionnaire* was remarkably complete and included citations to classical and current writings pertinent to each of the topics covered. Within a few years, however, the flood of new information from all over the world had grown almost beyond capture and the cost of production had more than doubled, so that only the large libraries could afford to buy the volumes.

A Common Language

Richet's fascination with the cataloguing of medical literature that stimulated him to create his *Bibliographica Physiologica* and his multivolume *Dictionnaire de Physiologie* also made him aware of the need for a common vehicle for communication, a universal language. He was attracted to Esperanto, invented by Ludwik Lejzer Zamenhof (1859–1917) a Polish Jew living under Russian rule. His book, written from prison under a pseudonym, *Dr. Esperanto's International Language*, gave the language its name which means, "The one who hopes." Richet urged the use of Esperanto, not only as a means to facilitate communications among scholars and thus accelerate the progress of science and culture in general, but to foster understanding among nations toward ultimate peace. He considered Esperanto by no means a substitute for native languages, which Richet felt should be preserved at all cost, but as an additional common language to be learned by everyone. Richet added Esperanto eagerly to his repertoire of causes. He was soon able to read it but never learned to speak the language.

The Professor's Literary Activities

In 1891 Richet published a book of fables in verse entitled *Pour les Grands et les Petits* intended for the delight and edification of his children. It appeared in several illustrated editions.[R 294; 695] and was recognized in a special award by the Académie Française.

Included as an introduction to the deluxe edition of *Pour les Grands et les Petits*, illustrated by Raphael Drouart[R 695] was the following poem:

Mon fils, si par hasard quelque vieillard tres vieux,
Etait un soir, par toi, recontré sur ta route,
Penchant sa tête lasse, et portant en ses yeux
Les voiles précurseurs de l'ombre qu'il redoute,
Ne sois pas trop cruel pour sa faiblesse, enfant.
Il n'est pas généraux d'être aussi triomphant,
Et de passer, superbe et hautain, sans rien dire,
Sans faire au pauvre aieul l'aumône d'un sourire.
Oui! ton aurore est belle et ton printemps en fleurs;
Tout est nouveau, vivant, plein de joie et de charmes;

Un papillion suffit pour dissiper tes pleurs,
Et tu ne connais pas l'amertume des larmes . . .
Mais lui, vois donc ces mains tremblantes, et ce front
Ridé par la source de la misère humaine!
Il connait la douleur, et le doute, et l'affront;
Et le remords peut-être, et l'angoissante peine;
Et les nuits sans sommeil, et les jours sans éspoir;
Et les écoeurements des laches servitudes;
Et les êtres chéris qu'on ne peut plus revoir;
Et les regrets, toujours plus poignants et plus rudes;
Mon fils! sois bon pour lui! La pitié, c'est beaucoup.
Beauté, vaillance, amour, jeunesse, ardente flamme,
Tous ces rayons divins du ciel ne sont pas tout;
Il faut y mettre encore un peu de grandeur d'âme . . .
Et puis, être clément, c'est être sage aussi.
Ce vieillard qui chancelle et tremble, c'est ton frère,
Et ce spectacle affreux qui t'épouvante ici,
C'est le sort qui t'attend. Rien ne peut t'y soustraire.
Un jour, ainsi qui lui, tu courberas le front,
Et quand, aux soirs d'été, menant joyeuse fête,
Les jeunes fous rieurs près de toi passeront,
Alors tu hocheras, morne, ta vielle tête.
A des déclins pareils tout être est condamné,
Marchant d'un pas fatal vers la froide vieillesse;
Le temps, qui ronge tout, le ronge pièce à pièce,
Déja presque un cadavre au moment qu'il est né.
La jeunesse et l'amour, c'est un rêve qui passe.
C'est un point dans le temps, comme un point dans
l'éspace.
Va! Crois-moi! c'est tenter la colère des cieux
Que d'être, ô mon cher fils, sans pitié pour les vieux.

* * *

My son, if perchance you should meet a very old man,
His head bent forward, his eyes veiled in shadows,
Do not scorn his feeble mein, my son.
To vaunt your triumph is ungenerous.
Don't pass him by in hauty silence
Without the favor of a smile, a precious gift.
Yes, your dawning is sublime, your spring in flower,
Your world is new, vibrant and full of joy.
A butterfly suffices to staunch your tears.
But he—his hands trembling and his forehead
Wrinkled by the strain of human misery!

He knows sorrow, doubt and humiliation
And remorse, perhaps, and anguished pain
And nights without sleep and days without hope
And the disheartening sense of servitude
And the thoughts of loved ones to be seen no more
and regrets more poignant, more burdensome with age.
My son, be good to him. Compassion is his due.
Your beauty, courage, love and youth,
All those gifts of heaven don't suffice.
A generous spirit must be added too.
To be gentle is also to be wise.
This trembling aging human is your brother
And in the autumn of your life
The young will jeer at you as you pass by.
You'll lower your old head in shame,
Walking toward the chill of helpless age.
Time erodes us all—and you as well.
Youth and love are dreams that quickly pass,
Just a point in time, a point in space.
Please believe. You tempt the rage of heaven,
My dear son, to show no pity for the old.

Apart from his books of poetry, Richet wrote novels and plays in verse. One, a successful dramatic play, *La Mort de Socrate*, was produced at the Odéon Theatre in Paris (1894). Another, *Circé*, was written a few years later. The idea for a short story, *Soeur Marthe*, occurred to Richet while attending the funeral of a friend. He had noted among the mourners "a very pale sick nun who sang with a touching voice." *Soeur Marthe* was well received, was later made into a novel, and finally into a libretto for a comic opera.[R410] Both *Circé* and *Soeur Marthe* tell a good deal about Richet's view of himself as a strong, proud, honorable, but sensitive, kind, and perceptive man. Both *Circé* and *Soeur Marthe* were written in verse. The protagonist in *Circé* is clearly Ulysses and in *Soeur Marthe* it is the naval officer Laurent, not Soeur Marthe herself. Both she and Circé were cast as lovelorn maidens who were longing for a man who was worthy in all respects, lordly, and sensitive. Such a man was Ulysses, proud and dignified, yet friendly and understanding with his men. His adequacy to meet Circé's sensuous demands was balanced by his singleness of purpose and high aspirations which finally caused him to leave her and return home. Richet's vision of the original myth ended with the death of Circé, unable to live without Ulysses.

The story of *Soeur Marthe* tells of a widely beloved and devout nun who, like Circé, becomes an irresistible temptress when the right man comes along. In this case it is Laurent, the brave, high-minded, dutiful naval officer who is kind enough to serve her longings. After what amounts to a bacchanal clothed in a hymnal, Soeur Marthe, too, dies as Laurent, heeding the higher call of duty, prepares to sail away.

In 1913 the Académie Française offered a prize for a poem in memory of Louis Pasteur. The entries were submitted anonymously. Richet's poem, "La Gloire de Pasteur" won the prize.[R627] Not knowing the identity of the winner, the judges asked a member of the Académie des Sciences to check the poem for technical accuracy. They were amazed to learn that their choice for the prize had recently been elected a member of the Académie des Sciences.

The judges requested that Richet remove from the poem his reference to the German scientists, Robert Koch and Paul Ehrlich. Richet agreed only to add lines that identified them as students of Pasteur, "making their work, therefore become a fragment of his glory." The judges also objected to Richet having referred to five- or six-day-old microbes as "ancient," but Richet refused to change the word.[16] The poem was never given a public reading, much to the disgust and anger of Pasteur's son-in-law René Vallery-Radot. Richet split the prize money between the towns of Dole, where Pasteur was born, and Arbois where he grew up.

Notes

1. Chaussier was appointed to the chair of anatomy and physiology at the Ecole de Santé established in 1795 upon the reopening of institutions that had been abolished in the wake of the French Revolution.
2. Richet was among those who were outraged when false evidence came to light in the conviction of Captain Alfred Dreyfus for espionage. He sent his visiting card with a note of encouragement to Emile Zola who had published "J'accuse," a diatribe aimed at the judges who had acquitted Major Esterhazy against whom there was more substantial evidence than there had been against Dreyfus. Dreyfus, however, was condemned to Devil's Island and Zola was tried and convicted for libel. Fortunately he escaped to England.
3. Richet's grandson, Gabriel, reported the same experience during his fishing trips with his grandfather.
4. Later Victor Pachon did further work in Marey's laboratory where he became highly adept in graphic methods. With Marey he created a recording sphygmograph, an oscillometric device for measuring blood pressure in humans which became known

as Le Pachon. (Pachon 1912). Sir Thomas Brunton (1844-1916), a distinguished Scottish physician who introduced the use of nitrites in the treatment of angina pectoris, credited the sphygmograph for his ability to record the rise in pressure that accompanied anginal pain. Indeed it was the rise in blood pressure that accompanies anginal pain that suggested to him the use of vasodilating nitrites (Fye 1986). While Pachon's instrument was superseded by the sphygmomanometer for measuring blood pressure, it is still used for directing circulatory impairment of the legs.

5. Three years later (1897) the first successful gastrectomy on a human was done by Carl Schlatter (1864-1934) on a patient with a diffuse gastric cancer. The woman was studied by Hoffman and Wroblewski. Hoffman found that she was able to deaminate ingested proteins normally and manufacture serum proteins as well (Hoffman 1898). Fat digestion, however, was less well performed without a stomach. Wroblewski in examining the woman's excreta found little disturbance attributable to the absence of HCl. Indeed, her vomitus contained lactic acid and her urine, too was strongly acidic. She died of disseminated cancer fourteen months after her operation (Wroblewski 1898).

6. In 1897 Walter Bradford Cannon (1871-1945), while still a medical student at Harvard and only two years after Wilhelm Konrad Röntgen's (1845-1923) discovery of x-ray, devised a way to visualize the stomach and record its contractions on x-ray film. While working with fellow student, Albert Moser, he fed a radio-opaque suspension of barium to animals and ultimately to humans. The ingested metallic fluid outlined the stomach and revealed its various shapes during contraction.

7. She and her family had prospered in the iron, steel, and coal business for generations. A great aunt of hers had wanted to marry James Buchanan, who later became president of the United States, but her father, thinking him beneath her, refused permission. She thereupon killed herself.

8. Richet anticipated, in a sense, modern knowledge of the control of membrane transport by relative ionic affinities. It was at about this time that the Swedish chemist, Svante August Arrhenius (1859-1927) discovered ionization for which he was awarded the Nobel Prize in 1902.

9. Quoted by Roux to Richet and freely translated, "I care not for the prizes, but only for their cash value." (Unp.)

10. Evidences of serum sickness, first recognized in 1905 by Clemens von Pirquet (1874-1929), an Austrian pediatrician who coined the term allergy and who served for a time as professor of pediatrics at Johns Hopkins Medical School in Baltimore, and by Bela Schick (1877-1967), a Hungarian pediatrician who became director of pediatrics at Mt. Sinai Hospital in New York.

11. Aufderheide and others have observed that, when cilia of paramecia are transposed experimentally and headed the wrong way, subsequent generations retain the transposed position with the cilia beating in the wrong direction. The apparent implication is that some inherited characteristics may not be controlled by the germ cell's nucleus.

12. A method of classifying elements by their atomic weight devised by Russian chemist Dmitri Ivanovich Mendeleev (1834-1907).

13. Eleven years later Wilbur Wright (1887-1912) wrote his famous letter to the Smithsonian Institution that stated, "I believe that simple flight, at least, is possible for man." Wright was proposing an instrument with fixed rather than flapping wings. He and his brother, Orville (1871-1948) constructed a biplane, however, not a monoplane as Richet and Tatin had.

14. Antoine Breguet was the fourth generation son of a remarkable family of Swiss engineers, inventors and clock and watchmakers. In 1774 Abraham-Louis Breguet established a home and business in the Quai de l'Horloge in Paris, a location that has remained in the Breguet family for more than 200 years. Each generation was able to adapt the Breguet talent to a rapidly developing new technology. Toward the end of the eighteenth-century, they contributed to the early development of automatic watches, new metallurgic processes in the manufacture of steel, marine chronometers, instruments for measuring electrical current, and they produced the first circuit breaking safety fuse. In the early nineteenth-century, they fashioned aneroid barometers and laboratory instruments for rapidly expanding French experimental science, and in the late nineteenth-century, railway controls, dynamos, and telephones. Finally, after the turn of the century, thanks to the experience of Louis and Jacques with Richet, they began the manufacture of airplanes and helicopters (Breguet 1980).

15. Calloier, literally a Greek monk of the order of St. Basile, but colloquially applied as "beau Vieillard," or fine old man. The word appears in a fourteenth-century poem by Eustache Deschamps.

16. In published versions of the poem the names of Koch and Ehrlich did not appear and neither is there a reference to ancient microbes.

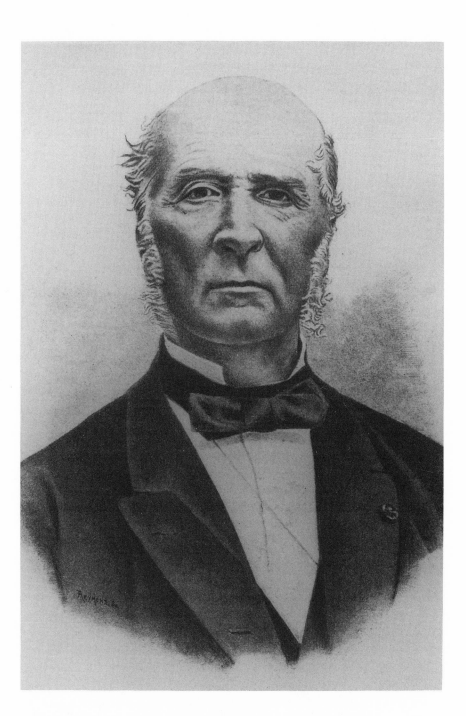

Charles Richet's father, Alfred (1816-1891) professor of surgery (1864-1887).

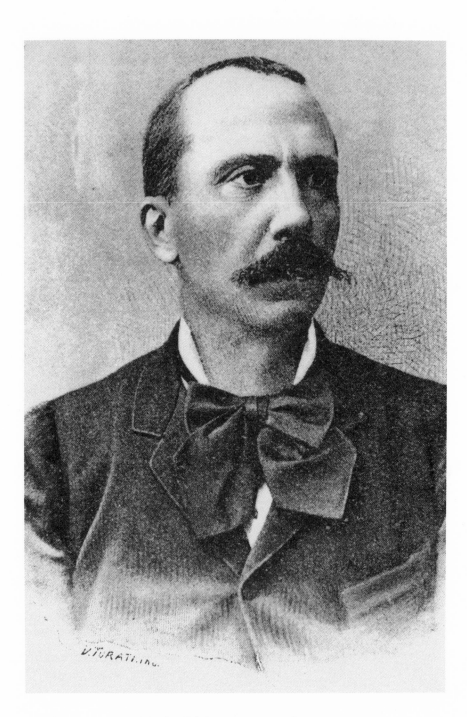

Charles Richet as a young doctor.

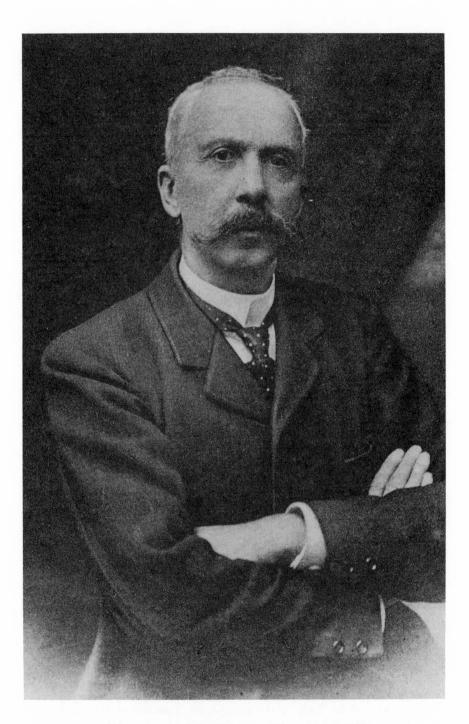

Charles Richet (1850-1935) professor of physiology (1887-1925).

The Oracle Speaks, caricature of Charles Richet [1913]. "The professional secret is an alluring fetish, but not one for which human lives should be sacrificed." [Richet refers to the prevailing legal requirement for confidentiality concerning everything about a patient, thereby preventing a physician from disclosing a patient's disease such as syphilis or tuberculosis to protect a family against infection].

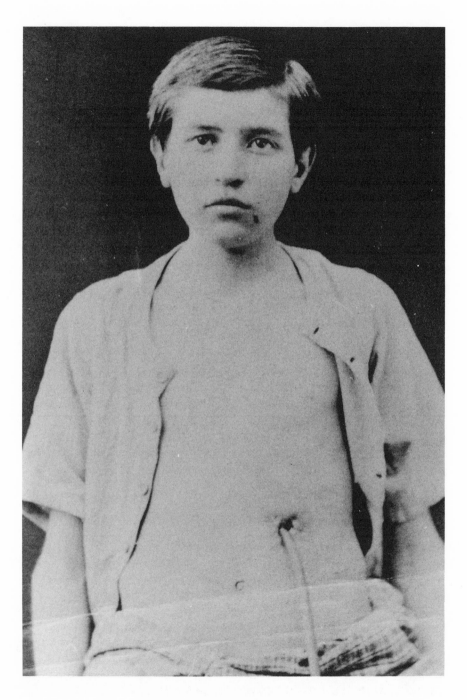

**Richet's subject, Marcellin, the young man with an opening through the
abdominal wall into his stomach.**

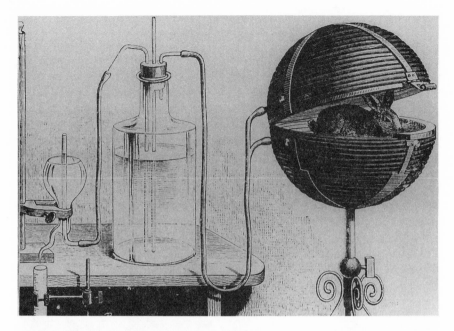

The siphon calorimeter devised by Richet (Courtesy of Comptes rendus de la Société de Biologie, February 6, 1885).

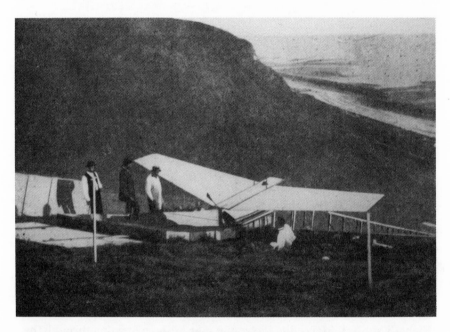

Richet (center left, standing behind Tatin) during early experiments on powered flight at Cap La Hève, 1890.

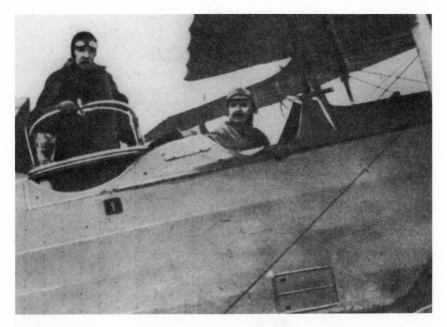

Richet (left) and Louis Bréguet preparing for takeoff in their gyroplane (early helicopter) in 1923.

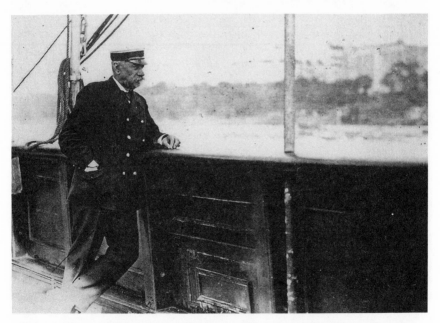

Prince Albert of Monaco on the deck of his marine biology yacht, the *Princesse Alice*, where Richet and Portier did their first experiments leading to the discovery of anaphylaxis. (Courtesy of Musée Oceanograhique de Monaco).

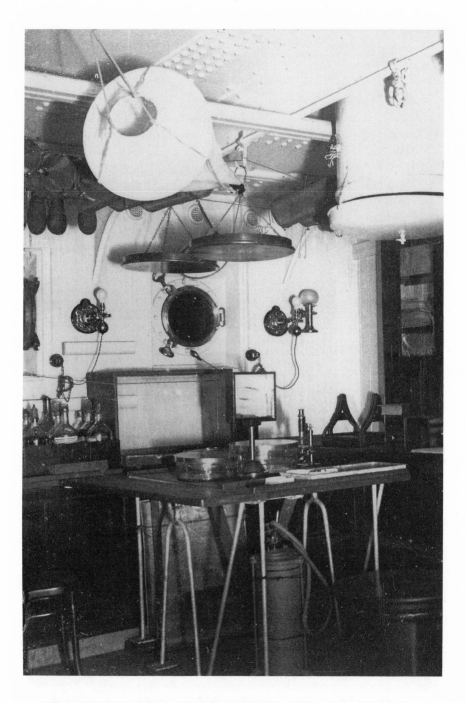

Research laboratory of the *Princesse Alice*. (Courtesy of Musée Oceanographique de Monaco).

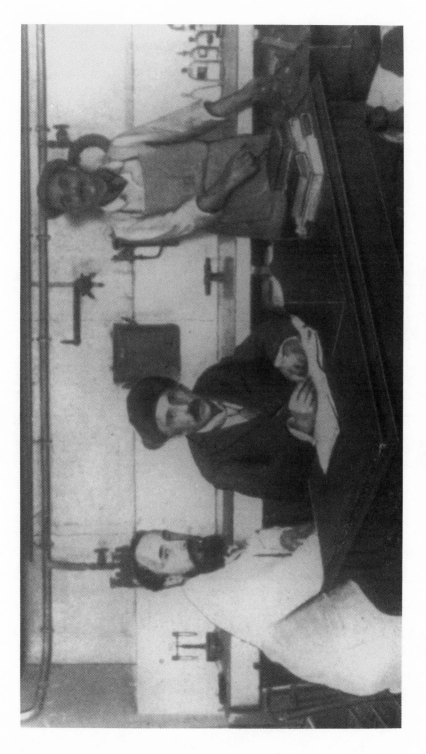

Richet in his own laboratory at work on anaphylaxis.

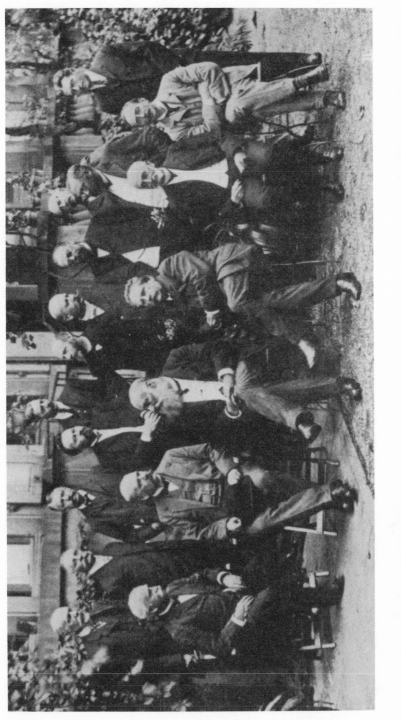

Richet at a gathering of distinguished members of the International Congress of Physiology including five Nobel Prize winners (Courtesy of Dr. Hubert Larcher).

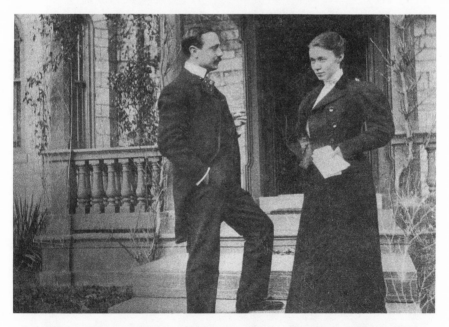

Toutes mes félicitations pour votre grand courage. Quoi qu'en

Charles Richet

Professeur à la Faculté de Médicine de Paris

dieut des égarés, nous êtes le défenseur de l'honneur de la France ; car l'honneur de la France, c'est la justice.

Charles Richet.

A note of congratulation and encouragement from Richet to Emile Zola whose famous article, "J'Accuse" had just appeared in Georges Clemenceau's newspaper *L'Auraure*.

Joachim and Anna Coleman Carvallo, one-time students of Richet, who originated the legislation for historic homes (Demeures Historiques) (Courtesy of Mr. Robert Carvallo).

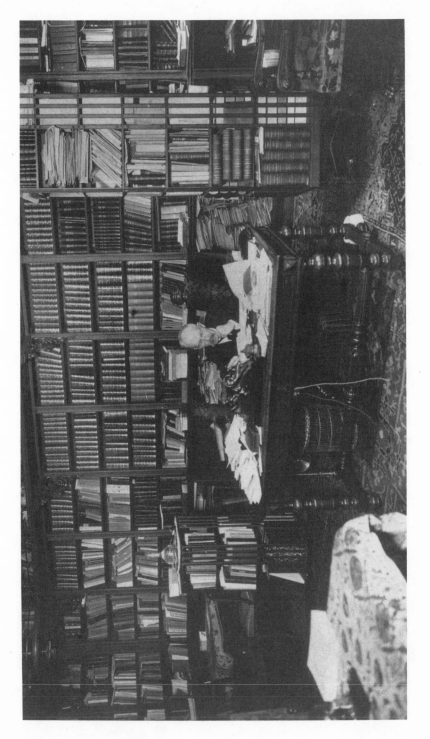

Richet seated in his beloved library.

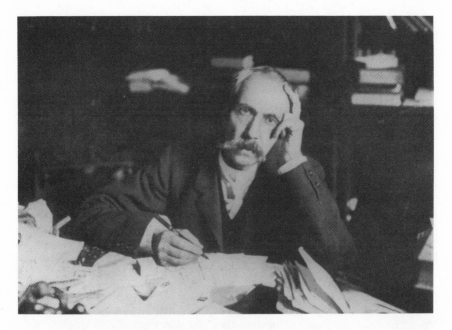

Charles Richet, 1909. The Pacifist-Patriot at work on *Le Passé de la guerre et l'avenir de la paix* (The end of war and the dawn of peace).

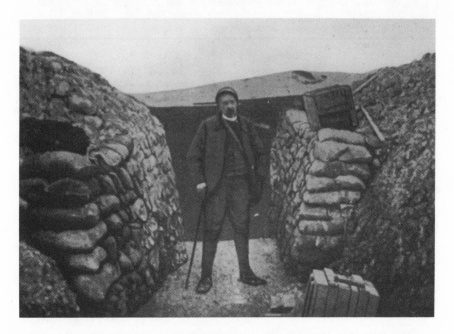

Richet in the trenches in World War I (1917). The pioneer of plasma transfusion.

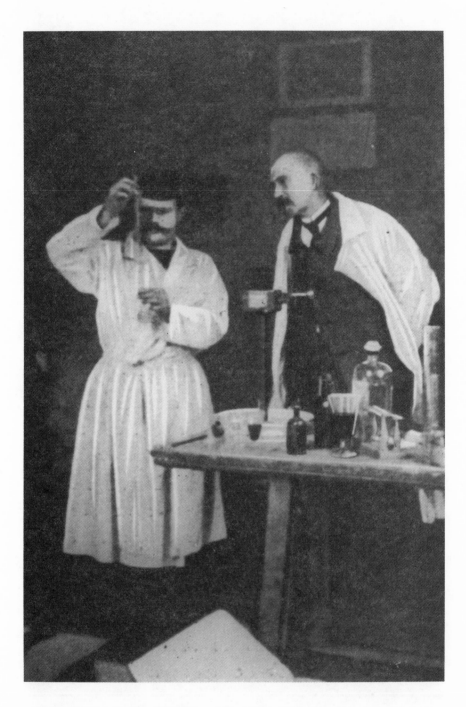

Charles Richet in his ambulance laboratory in the combat zone between Reims and Soissons. Winter of 1918.

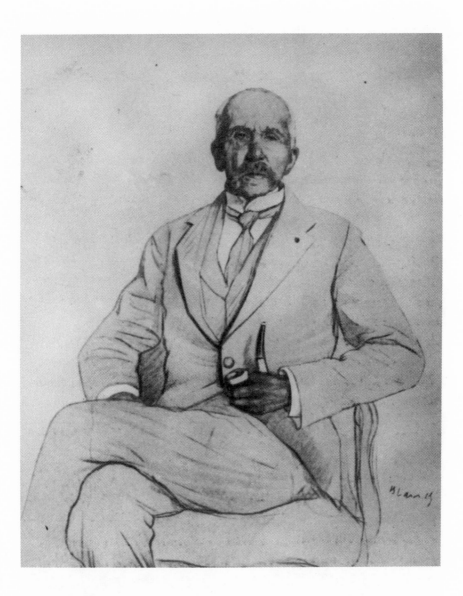

A painting of Richet at his retirement after 38 years as professor.

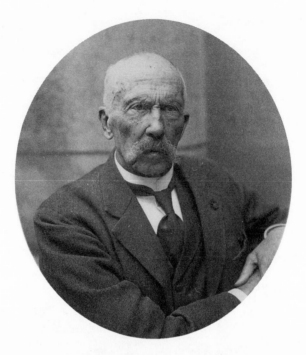

Near the end. A photograph dedicated to a distinguished friend (Courtesy of Dr. Hubert Larcher).

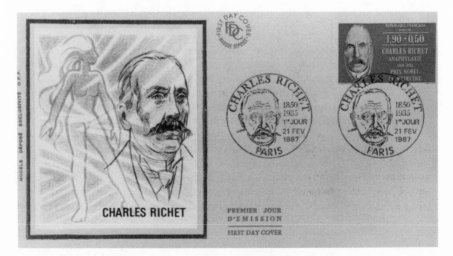

A commemorative stamp and envelope issued on the centenary of Richet's appointment as professor.

6

Achievement and Acclaim 1902–1914

In a characteristic way Richet's love of travel became entangled with his literary and scientific endeavors in an adventure from which his most important contribution to physiology emerged. Paul Régnard, his colleague at the Marine Biology Laboratory at Le Havre and close friend of Prince Albert of Monaco, suggested to Richet that he ask the prince for permission to join him on a cruise of his research yacht, the *Princesse Alice*. When Richet approached the prince he was welcomed despite his having no special project in mind. The prince suggested that Richet and another physiologist on board, Paul Portier (1866–1962), *agrégé* and later professor of physiology at the Sorbonne, study the venom of the pneumatocysts of the *Physalia*, or Portugese man-o-war. Richet, who had been interested in poisons since his student days, readily agreed. What seemed to him a pleasant, diversionary experience led Richet to the Nobel Prize and sparked nearly two centuries of rapid progress in uncovering the dark mysteries of the human immune system.

The yacht set sail from Toulon with Prince Albert in charge on 5 July 1901. For the first few weeks of the voyage fishing was poor and there were no Portugese men-o-war in evidence. Meanwhile, Richet passed the time completing *Circé* a tragic drama in verse about a colorful incident in the travels of Homer's hero Ulysses. Richet read the play to Prince Albert who was so pleased with it that he had it produced at the Théatre de Monte Carlo on 2 April 1905 with Sarah Bernhardt in the title role.[1] The play was published in 1920 with the following dedication to Prince Albert: "During the clear nights aboard your yacht in the equatorial Atlantic, I told you of my dream which, thanks to you, became a reality in one of the most sumptuous theaters in the world where an admirable and genial artiste gave to 'Circé' her eloquence, her passion, her beauty, and despair. Thank you most respectfully. Charles Richet."

As the *Princesse Alice* neared the Cape Verde Islands the men-o-war finally appeared. Richet set up a plan to study the beasts based on his earlier work in which repeated exposure of bacteria to metallic salts yielded eventual immunity to the poison. Richet, therefore, thought that it might be possible to adapt animals and man to the effects of poisons, by initially injecting an extremely small quantity of the substance and then gradually increasing the dose. After extracts of the pneumatocysts had been filtered through sand, the glycerinated bluish fluid was injected into pigeons, ducks, guinea pigs and frogs. The first pigeon injected promptly became comatose, so much so that when he was attacked by a parrot, who removed part of the skin of his head, he made no movement and gave no evidence of discomfort. As the cruise ended Portier and Richet agreed to continue their collaboration back in France.

On their return to Paris they resumed their investigation but were unable to find an adequate supply of *Physalia*. They, therefore, turned to actinia (sea anemones), which they found in profusion among the rocks along the seashore at Carqueiranne and at Roscoff in Brittany. The tentacles of actinia were found to contain a powerful vascular congestant that was quickly fatal to rabbits and other small animals. A comparable dose given to dogs produced very little reaction. Léon René Binet (1893–1966) quoted the following from what he stated was Richet's *cahier d'expériences* (laboratory notebook):

Neptune [the name of a dog] on 14 January 1902 received 0.05 cc/kg of actinotoxin. One hour after this weak dose the dog walked about the laboratory in good spirits. January 17: To see if this dog was sensitized, we injected him with 0.1 cc/kg; again there was no untoward reaction. January 18: The dog is not sick and appears in good spirits. We were too close to the first injection. February 10: The dog is in perfect health, active with glistening coat. At 14 hours he was injected with 0.12 cc/kg of toxin. Immediately there followed vomiting, defecation, trembling of the forelimbs and the dog fell on his side unconscious. One half hour later he was dead. The dog was literally overwhelmed by this second injection which could have caused a fresh dog only mild discomfort. The dog has offered us a striking spectacle which has dispelled any doubts we might have had. Not only were animals repeatedly injected with weak doses of toxin at the correct time not immunized, but were certainly sensitized. This new phenomenon merited a special name. We gave it the name anaphylaxis, from the Greek word *phylaxis* protection, joined to the prefix *ana*, contrary to.[R 426] February 19, 1902: "A substance insufficient to kill or even sicken a normal animal produces fulminating symptoms and death in an animal previously inoculated with the same substance. (Binet 1952)

It seems likely that the lines that Binet quoted were taken from notes for a presentation rather than from data recorded as the experiments were being carried out. As noted above, his hypothesis on undertaking the experiments was not that animals might be sensitized, but rather, that they might be adapted to the effects of poisons by initially injecting an extremely small dose of the substance and subsequently administering gradually increasing doses. In the note quoted by Binet, Richet refers to the third injection as the second. Moreover the dosage figures differed from those recalled by Richet as he dictated his *Souvenirs d'un Physiologiste* to his grandson - 0.1 gm/kg in the first injection, 0.1 gm/kg three weeks later. Likewise the published paper that appeared shortly afterward in the *Comptes Rendus* of that society, states that Neptune received only two identical doses, 0.1 gm/kg on two occasions three weeks apart.

Richet and Portier promptly established that Neptune's death was not due to the direct effect of the poison. They found that giving a second injection to animals within a few hours, or even five days after the first one did not produce the dramatic fatal outcome, as it had also apparently failed to do in Neptune after an interval of three days. Thus, as Richet reasoned, there must be a period of incubation. He and Portier did further experiments with a variety of substances and found that, when a second injection of the same substance was given approximately three weeks after the first, symptoms identical with those of Neptune occurred and overshadowed or replaced whatever pharmacological effects might have been expected from the substance itself.

Other scientists had observed the phenomenon before the work of Richet and Portier but had not studied it systematically. One was Magendie, referred to by Richet in his article on immunity in his *Dictionnaire de Physiologie:* "Magendie in 1839 had noted that the first injection of egg albumin into an animal caused no disturbance but a second injection, given a few days later to the same animal, proved lethal (Magendie 1839). Also von Behring, Knorr and others who injected animals with diphtheria and tetanus toxins to prepare antitoxins found that repeated injection might produce illness or death. Such poorly understood findings were variously interpreted, even being attributed to errors in technique."[R 544] Richet's close friend Victor Clarence Vaughan (1851-1929) had also noted the phenomenon. To save money on his studies of antipneumococcus serum he had obtained from the Lilly Company "used" rabbits already immunized against the pneumococcus. He was dismayed to find that most of them died promptly after his first injection of serum but he failed to appreciate the significance of what he had seen (Vaughan 1926).

A note filed in the Archives of the Oceanographic Museum of Monaco, not dated, but presumably written in 1910 or 1911 by Dr. Richard who had been present on the cruise of the *Princesse Alice*, recounts the transition of Richet's thoughts from the hypnotoxin, produced by *Physalia*, to anaphylaxis observed in the actinia experiments and then to immunity (Richard 1910).

By 1906 Portier, having decided not to continue studying the phenomenon, had returned to his responsibilities at the Sorbonne. In his *Mémoires* Richet praised Portier for "giving up all claim to the honor of the discovery.[2] In 1907 Richet, using an extract from hura crepitans, a poisonous plant that he had found on a trip to Brazil, demonstrated that susceptibility to anaphylaxis could be transferred from one animal to another by injecting the serum of an animal that had received an injection of a poison into a second animal that had received no poison injection. Richet demonstrated that blood serum from the animal previously injected with the poison produced anaphylaxis on the first injection into the second animal. From these observations Richet concluded that an innate mechanism, presumably in the central nervous system, must serve as the mediator of anaphylaxis.[R 501] [3] In another important experiment conducted in 1909, Richet showed that mixing in vitro the serum from a sensitized animal with the substance that had initially induced the sensitivity, produced anaphylaxis upon its injection into a new animal.[R 501] He further discovered that an animal that had managed to recover from anaphylaxis would thenceforth be immune to the dose of the substance responsible for anaphylaxis. Richet reasoned from these observations that anaphylaxis must involve an antitoxin in the blood of the animal, presumably as a protection against a foreign substance.[4] For these seminal investigations of sensitivity and immunity Richet was awarded the Moscow Prize at the International Physiological Congress in London in 1912.

Richet's discovery of anaphylaxis with its seeming relevance to immunity had enlarged the field of immunology beyond microbes and had set off an intense flurry of activity among investigators in Europe and America. Most immunologists found the idea that the selfsame substance could act as a sensitizer and immunizer difficult to encompass. They found the mechanisms involved in hypersensitivity and immunity even more baffling. Although anaphylaxis appeared to most to be related to immunity, it was not clear whether or not it was a necessary stage toward achieving immunity. Tackling the problem with a variety of protein-aceous substances in different amounts and with differing techniques most workers concluded that the initial injection caused a sensitizing (and immunizing) substance to be formed in the body but they conceived of it differently and called it by various names.

Their findings reinforced Richet's inference from his earlier work on serotherapy that immunizing substances are produced by the invaded body itself, not by the invading agent. This view was contrary to that of Pasteur, discussed in chapter 5 that immunity is acquired because the first invasion by an organism either depletes the tissues of the host of some factor essential to the bacteria's growth or adds new substances that inhibit its subsequent growth (Dubos 1950). Pasteur's concept had already yielded to the discovery by Metchnikoff (1901) of the capacity of white blood cells to engulf and destroy bacteria (phagocytosis) and to Paul Ehrlich's discovery of an antibacterial substance in the blood of immunized individuals (Ehrlich 1897).

The sequence of studies that uncovered and to some extent integrated the complicated serological behavior responsible for anaphylaxis were reviewed up to 1908 in a lecture to the Harvey Society by Anderson and Rosenau (1909). They acknowledged the tentative nature of their inter-pretations but predicted that "a final solution of the mechanism of anaphylaxis will have a practical application in the treatment and pre-vention of a number of disease dates."

Other prominent contributors were Maurice Arthus (1862–1945); Alexander Besredka (1870–1940), who was largely responsible for working out the process of desensitization (Besredka 1911, 1916); Paul Ehrlich; Charles Jules Henri Nicolle (1866–1936); John Auer (1875–1948), who found that anaphylactic shock could be prevented by prior administration of atropine (Auer 1910); Theobald Smith (1859–1934); Victor Vaughan and Frederick Parker Gay (1874–1939).

Richet involved anaphylaxis in his concept of defense of the organism. As such it accelerated progress toward the concept of a natural immune system, protective against all manner of foreign substances. Although, as pointed out by Moulin, the use of the actual phrase "immune system" awaited the development of cellular immunology in the 1960s (Moulin 1989). In her beautifully reasoned synthesis Moulin shows how the phagocytic, humoral, and cellular theories of immunity were unified and recognized as regulatory functions of the central nervous system and, in the adaptive evolutionary sense, of genetics as well. The ultimate integration stemmed from the conceptual contributions of Elie Metchnikoff (1845–1916) as developed by his pupil Besredka and a trail of other contributions.

In 1902, within a few months of the initial publication of Portier and Richet, Maurice Arthus of Lausanne embarked on a systematic long-term study of anaphylaxis. He showed that nonpoisonous substances, including blood serum, could produce anaphylaxis and added important new clinically significant features, including one that bears his name (Arthus 1921).[5] Having made his initial discovery of anaphylaxis with poison, Richet had continued to consider anaphylaxis as peculiar to poisonous substances until the work of Arthus. Arthus repeatedly emphasized this point in his book, urging that his discovery of the anaphylactic effect of serum be known as the Arthus Phenomenon and Richet's finding of the effect of repeated injections of poison be identified separately as the Richet Phenomenon (Arthus 1921).

In 1906 M.J. Rosenau and John F. Anderson (1873–1958) added the important discovery that the anaphylactic state may be induced by extremely small doses of a variety of foreign proteins including egg white (Rosenau, Anderson 1906). The contributions of Arthus (Sigerist 1943) and Rosenau and Anderson (1902) confirmed and extended Richet's finding that anaphylaxis was not attributable to the nature of the inciting agent itself but to a specific reaction in the body to a subsequent exposure to any one of a variety of agents, the initial administration of which had been harmless. It appeared that the reaction required some sort of chemical combination within the body but the nature of the substances (antigen-antibody) and the mode of action of their combination was a matter of dispute.

Anaphylaxis had offered Richet an opportunity to reexamine his experiments on immunity. He had predicted that because the manifestations of anaphylaxis were so widespread and included bronchospasm, hypotension, bloody vomitus, and diarrhea, that the trigger for the symptom complex would be found in the central nervous system. Like so many of his shrewd insights, this one proved to be correct. In addition, however, Richet had recognized the connection between anaphylaxis and immunity since he had demonstrated that animals that survived an anaphylactic shock were thenceforth immune to the offending substance. It was not until very recent years, however, that research on immunology turned to the nervous system where Richet had thought that it should be directed. Now it is generally recognized that the entire widely distributed and complex immune system with its cellular, humoral and hormonal messages is ultimately under the control of the brain (Raine 1988).

A Festschrift with International Participation

In May 1912 the Académie de Médecine held a symposium and reception in honor of Richet's twenty-five years as professor. The sixty-four presentations by physiologists from several countries were ultimately published by the Imprimerie de la Cour d'Appel in 1912 in a handsome volume called *Mélanges Biologiques*.[R 534] Appendix 6.1 lists the contributors and their topics. Maurice Arthus reported his studies on the capability of nontoxic proteins to produce anaphylaxis; Fernand Widal, another prominent scientist whose work was stimulated by Richet's discovery of anaphylaxis, described autoanaphylaxis resulting from reinjection of the patients' own previously stored blood; André Broca spoke of the anatomy and physiology of the retina. The Belgian physiologist Paul Heger (1864-1925) presented new data on the effect of altitude on the heart. Ivan Pavlov, famous for his work on conditional reflexes, described internal inhibition in relation to the structure of the two hemispheres of the brain. It was his first publication of that material in other than the Russian language. Charles Sherrington, the British neurophysiologist already mentioned and, like Ivan Pavlov, a Nobel laureate, presented a reflective history of neurophysiology. He credited Richet's demonstration of "antagonistic" muscles in the claw of crayfish with the initial recognition of the essential role of inhibition in any useful movement of an extremity. Further in his discussion, Sherrington acknowledged Richet's contribution to the recognition of a refractory state in the central as well as peripheral nervous system. The French physician-chemist Armand Gautier's (1837-1920) paper examined the process of scientific creativity that leads to discovery. He cited the work of Henri Poincaré (1854-1912), Louis Pasteur, Claude Bernard, Lavoisier, Christopher Columbus (1451-1506), and others. He concluded with what appeared to be an appreciative "tip of the hat" to Richet: "those who were guided only by fact and logic doubtless contributed to discoveries, but the intuitive spirits have planted the fields where their predecessors had labored and thereupon have gathered the richest harvest." Other contributors to the symposium included the British physiologist, William Maddock Bayliss (1860-1924) who spoke on energy consumption of sustained contraction of muscles being less than that associated with repeated contractions, and Maurice Mendelssohn who demonstrated electrical phenomena in the movement of leukocytes. Only one of the papers presented at the symposium dealt with Richet's beloved field of metapsychology, J.E. Abelous, his former fellow and colleague, now a professor at the Faculté de Médecine in Toulouse, reported on extrasensory perception.

Adolph Pinard, professor of obstetrics of the Faculté de Médecine dealt with another of Richet's favorite topics, eugenics. He attributed the origin of the idea of perfecting the human race to Francis Bacon and Condorcet, adding that Darwin's revelation of natural selection finally established the feasibility of achieving such perfection as proposed in Richet's book *La Sélection Humaine*, which Pinard had an opportunity to read in manuscript. Pinard went on to endorse Richet's radical proposal of controlled human breeding that urged the widespread distribution of the genes of geniuses, civilized Western Europeans and savants such as himself toward the creation of a superior race of men. Pinard, the founder of the Société Française Eugenique in 1912 had previously been an exponent of a much milder program to improve the human race, puericulture, the attentive care of pregnant women and their offspring, especially during the early years (Schneider 1986a).[6]

Richet's Involvement in Eugenics

The book, *La Sélection Humaine*, which, as noted above, Pinard had read in manuscript in 1912, was not to appear until 1919, the year Richet was elected vice president of the Société Française Eugénetique. At that time Richet had already formulated his concept of defense of the organism which, as described in his 1893 article in *Revue Scientifique*, his 1894 text book and the 1902 volume of *Dictionnaire de Physiologie*, did not include eugenics. Nevertheless, he found no difficulty incorporating it in his overall formulation of defense of the family, the nation, and the human race.

Sir Francis Galton (1822-1911), anthropologist and cousin of Charles Darwin and well known for his studies of identical twins coined the term *eugenics* and is generally credited with being the founder of the science.

He was interested in socially controllable factors that would either improve or impair the qualities of future generations. Others interested in the potential of human breeding and selective sterilization included Charles Eliot, president of Harvard, Winston Churchill, and Beatrice and Sidney Webb (Degler 1990). Growing public interest led to the establishment in California of a sperm bank to reproduce the genes of Nobel Prize winners and "geniuses." After World War I, Darwinian sociology had begun to lose adherents as a popular preoccupation with "nurture" began to replace that of "nature." According to Carl Degler, the suppression of genetic thinking began with political pressures that promoted the idea of the equality of the races, the emergence of behavioral psychology with John B. Watson (1878–1958) and Burrhus Frederic Skinner (1904–1991), the philosophical and social teachings of John Dewey (1859–1952), George Herbert Mead (1863–1931) and William Isaac Thomas (1863–1947) and such anthropologists as Franz Boas (1858–1942).

There was a brief revival of interest in eugenics during the worldwide depression of the 1930s as the French were competing for jobs with North African immigrants, but not until after World War II did the sociobiologists reappear and refocus the attention of social scientists on the genetic basis of temperament and talent.

In the interval, however, Richet maintained his point of view that he had recorded in 1912. In a sense his commitment to eugenics represented the culmination of a long and deep concern with the quality of humanity and the future of Europe. The following somewhat scattered quotations from *La Sélection Humaine* illustrate the depth of Richet's feelings:

Happiness is the goal, wrote Richet, happiness and justice, not just for ourselves but for all humans. Our ancestors have willed us riches of all sorts. We must add to them. We are surrounded by enemies, the weather, sickness, and our own vices. Only knowledge through science and its application can attenuate human misery. One feels complete joy only in rare moments when one is very young. Joy is fleeting. The sense of suffering is more persistent. One must improve the human race by breeding as one does animals and plants. Marriage has become a social function rather than a natural function, thus interfering with the operation of selection for the strongest and most intelligent with no concern for personal qualities and less for posterity. We should breed toward a noble spirit and a beautiful body. Civilization, which has done so much for the benefit of the individual, will yield only degradation of the human species. The aristocracy is evidence of the genetic superiority of some families and they are properly given certain privileges. Intelligence has not evolved, only the means by which to use it. If humans should be bred for intelligence, intelligence would probably increase. Specialization inhibits intellectual development. One must eliminate the causes of deterioration from alcohol by preventing its sale; tuberculosis by removing the patient to Ireland, Corsica, the Philippines, Sardinia, Crete, and Ceylon. First of all one must avoid all mixture of superior races with the inferior. Whites are superior to blacks because they are more intelligent and we know that from an experiment of nature. The blacks have not produced an Archimedes (287 B.C. - 212 B.C.) or a Pasteur. Booker T. Washington cannot balance Virgil, Voltaire (François Marie Arouet 1694-1778), etc. The Chinese have done nothing for the historical, social, or linguistic sciences. Their law is common, uncouth; in which torture plays the preponderant role. Their language is prodigiously bizarre and incoherent. The Chinese literary and artistic works are far from being unimportant. Nevertheless, they have exerted very little influence on ours. My opinion in this regard is only personal. Who after all would dare establish immutable esthetic rules? Anyway, for my part, I would give the entire Chinese theater with its 25 million plays (which I have not read) for Hamlet and Oedipus; all of the Chinese philosophers including Confucius for the thoughts of Marcus Aurelius and the *Critique of Pure Reason*; all of the Chinese pagodas including the Great Wall for the Parthenon and Sainte-Chapelle; all the paunchy Buddhas and grotesque Asiatics for the *Dying Gladiator*; all the screens, fans, porcelains, parasols; all the trinkets of the entire Celestial Empire for a painting by Rembrandt; and the cymbals, Chinese hats and cacophonies of the oriental world for a Beethoven symphony. I will repeat for the yellow races what I said before for the blacks; let us suppose that the planet earth contained only Europe and the Mediterranean Sea without vast Asia, without savage Africa. What aspect of humanity would have been less advanced? Without Asia and Africa we would have had Egypt, Greece, Rome, Italy, France, Germany, and England and the entire civilized world of today which, eager for liberty and knowledge, works valiantly toward the conquest of truth. Nothing would have been changed by the absence of the yellow race. We would not have lost either a theorem, an experiment, or a machine. We would have fewer vases. Our moral philosophy would have stayed the same because we owe it to Socrates (470-399) to Christ, to Marcus Aurelius, to Kant. The famous spirit of Buddha and the phantasmagories of the Vedas have happily contributed nothing. The idea of progress of the human race and of individual humans inspires our every action and directs our entire conduct. We would be taking the wrong path if we allow ourselves to be contaminated by the men of the orient. Schools, telegraphs, and newspapers came from us and us alone. To conclude, since the proper criterion is intelligence, we must place at the bottom of the hierarchy of the human race the blacks who are incapable of thinking or innovating and are unable to constitute themselves as a nation. Very far above them we place the yellow race with little inventiveness or creativity but brave, hard working, and capable of learning quickly. Finally, way above, we place the white race which has accomplished the most in the world, has created the intelligent well-organized society, has invented thousands of industries, has used natural resources and animals at will, and has conquered through science the entire planet. These are neither theories nor fantasies; they are reality itself with all its resplendent brutality.

Like many of his contemporaries basically interested in human betterment, Richet could be said to have been blinded by the much exaggerated theories of "Darwinism," thus his text continues:

Marriages of whites with blacks or yellows should be prohibited by law. After having eliminated the inferior races one must eliminate deaf mutes and defective specimens.

Malformed infants should be killed at birth. Older defectives of all sorts should be prohibited marriage—castration in some instances. Just as it is reasonable to limit eligibility for military service, it is equally so in the case of marriage. There remain the illegitimate children, these wretched products of degraded parents who had been recognized as ineligible for marriage, born into terrible conditions, will have little chance of long life or fecundity. One has no right to marry if one is able only to have miserable children.

Richet concluded a lecture to the French Society of Eugenics with the words, "human selection will be the primary concern and the major effort of future generations."

Stockholm and the Nobel Prize

In the fall of 1912, the same year that the above quotations flowed from the pen of Charles Richet and two weeks after the wedding of his son Charles *fils*, Richet received a telegram announcing his selection for the Nobel Prize. "Before that I knew nothing about it," wrote Richet. "Shortly afterward, with my wife and some of my children, I made the voyage to Stockholm. I frequently joke with young people: 'If you would like to take a delightful trip, go receive the Nobel Prize in Stockholm.'" He recounted an incident at the award ceremony when the king presented him the medal. Being a little flustered Richet said, "Thank you, excellency" (instead of Your Majesty). A few moments later he saw the king and the princess laughing together. When the time came for Richet to escort the princess to the banquet, Richet offered her his arm and said, "you were making fun of me." "No," said the princess, "we were not making fun of you but we were laughing."[R736] Richet was impressed with her awareness of the fine distinctions of the French language.[7]

Richet's address at the presentation of the prize gave scant credit to Portier, the senior author of the original report who apparently had little interest in the work and withdrew as a collaborator before the studies were concluded. Nevertheless, at Richet's death, Portier succeeded to his place in the Académie des Sciences.

According to Henri Bouquet's commentary on Richet, published in 1935, Portier did not grasp the significance of the sudden catastrophic death of the dog Neptune after a second dose of poison from the tentacles of the sea anemone three weeks after the dog had survived the injection of a comparable dose without incident (Bouquet 1935).[8]

As impressive as were Richet's contributions to the study of immunity and other fields of research they were not recognized by the Académie des Sciences until he had won the Nobel Prize. He had applied several times before but each time was turned down in favor of another candidate. Among his successful opponents were Jacques Arsène d'Arsonval and Albert Dastre, both outstanding physiologists in the tradition of Claude Bernard; Charles Louis Alfonse Laveran (1845–1922), who had discovered the malaria parasite within red blood cells; and Marie Marcellin Lucas-Championière (1843–1913), a surgeon who had introduced antisepsis in France. It was on the death of the latter that in 1913 Richet was finally elected to a chair usually reserved for a surgeon. In 1933, two years before his death, Richet became president of the Académie des Sciences.

Appendix 6.1

TABLE DES MATIERES*

*Pour quelques-uns des mémoires composant cet ouvrage (voy. à la fin de la table), l'ordre alphabétique n'a pu être suivi, soit que ces mémoires eux-mêmes, soit que les épreuves corrigées aient été envoyés en retard par les auteurs.

Notes

1. After a successful series of performances of *Circé*, Bernhardt agreed to appear in Richet's play, *Possession*, but dropped the idea when her friend, the playwright Victorien Sardou, told her, "If you want to appear in a play about the occult, I have one ready for you." Despite the presence of the star, Sardou's play, called *Spiritisme*, was a failure.
2. Portier had joined the cruise of the Princesse Alice as a marine biologist. Although an M.D. and a professor of physiology, his work had dealt with marine animals and insects, especially butterflies. It is likely, therefore, that his interests were those of a naturalist rather than a medical scientist. Perhaps he sought answers in terms of "what is it like, what does it do and from what did it develop?" rather than the more medically oriented way of asking: "how does it work and how can it be modified?" If true, it is not difficult to understand his reluctance to continue with the study of anaphylaxis and his willingness to cede the credit to Richet.
3. The work on anaphylaxis soon attracted so much attention among investigators that Richet, redoubling his efforts to keep ahead, needed to expand the facilities of his dogs. Fortunately, Brouardel who was now dean, had established a laboratory annex for the medical faculty on the Boulevard Brune at the end of the rue de Vanves. Richet appropriated most of the space for his own research since very few of his faculty colleagues came to work there. "I could only assume," wrote Richet, "that their small quarters at the university were adequate for what work they were doing (Unp). Richet spent most of his time at the new facility experimenting with anaphylaxis and continuing his studies of zomotherapy and of lactic fermentation as well.
4. This idea had first occurred to Richet while he watched Pasteur, during a visit with Vulpian to Pasteur's laboratory. Using a culture of organisms grown repeatedly on artificial media, Pasteur demonstrated immunization of chickens to fowl cholera. The maneuver attentuated bacterial virulence so that, after causing only a mild illness, the injected animals were immunized to further exposure to the organism. Richet reasons that in response to the injected organisms the body must have produced some sort of chemical defense against subsequent infection.
5. The Arthus phenomenon is a local area of tissue destruction in a sensitized person induced by injection of a small dose of the appropriate antigen into the skin.
6. The word puericulture was first used in 1865 in a government instruction manual on the care of young children by the French physician Alfred Caron. The transition from puericulture to eugenics was influenced by the widespread attention to Darwin's *Origin of Species by Natural Selection* that appeared originally in 1859 (Darwin 1859).
7. "Non, nous ne sommes pas moqués, mais nous avons ri."
8. As already noted, Portier, as a marine biologist and entomologist, may have had interests in biology quite different from those of Richet, a medical scientist. Hence he may have had less curiosity about anaphylaxis than Richet and less understanding of its medical significance.

7

The Dedicated Pacifist and Patriot 1914–1925

Richet attributed his "abhorrence of war" to the influence of his grandfather, Charles Renouard, who had been a determined and vocal opponent of the Napoleonic Wars. Since age twenty, when he served as a hospital aide and ambulance attendant during the disastrous Franco-Prussian war, Richet had realized that war brings not only great suffering and destruction but disrupts productive intellectual intercourse among nations. Nevertheless in that war of 1870–71, during the Commune and even during World War I when he was in his late sixties, Richet, as a patriot, did not hesitate to expose himself to danger. Despite his record of valor, Richet, between the wars, committed himself to work for peace. As early as 1884 he had become a member of the Société de la Paix. He was also very active in the Société de l'Arbitrage entre Nations, later becoming its president. In 1900 he presided over the World Congress of Peace in Paris. He urged that ordinary citizens be given a greater voice in world affairs in order to moderate the vainglorious ambitions of rulers, politicians, and governments, and to counteract the chauvinistic, excitable, and often inflammatory writings that appeared in the press. As a man dedicated to the idea of "rights," he held the view that serious disputes among nations should be settled by the World Court at The Hague or by a similar body that had appropriate international representatives. He had dedicated his book, *Le Passé de la guerre et l'avenir de la paix*, published in 1907, to his grandfather Charles Renouard: "It was he who inspired my thoughts and consequently this book. It is he who taught me the two faces of war, ferocity and stupidity. It is he who from my earliest years gave me a love for blessed justice which nothing can suppress. What the elderly man has taught the child, the man in his prime should, in his turn, teach the young people."[R 488]

In the book Richet discussed the benefits of war over against its costs and losses and pointed out that on biologic, metaphysic, historic, moral, patriotic, and even opportunistic grounds war is not profitable. Weighing the strength of his arguments, he concluded, "Let us admit that in view of prevailing prejudices only a few [wars] will be avoided. Perhaps this sparing of blood will make the effort worthwhile."[R 488] The historian William Schneider reported that "When Richet received his Nobel Prize for physiology, the German pacifist Bertha von Suttner wrote him that he should have been awarded the Peace Prize instead" (Schneider 1986b). She had been present at the Congress of Physiology at Heidelberg and had heard Richet's remarks at the banquet. He wrote of it in his *Mémoires*:

> perhaps because of the generous offering of wine, I enjoyed true oratorical success.
> . . I felt inspired. I spoke of the war (1870) which for so long had torn apart Germany and France. I spoke of the destruction of the older part of Heidelberg, the atrocities of former times. I spoke of peace, holy, divine peace that allows men to work together, as we do, for a better destiny without seeking any recompense except to have made less arduous the lives of others. I quoted Goethe "Das Lied, das aus der Kehle dringt, ist Lohn der reichlich lohnt.[1] The entire audience rose, transported, I had responded that evening to the intimate feelings of each one. My wise colleague, Walter Kossel [1888-1956] of Heidelberg could only squeeze my hand with tears in his eyes and say "Herrlich, herrlich" [noble, noble]. Alas, it was only words but the remembrance of them will always live in my heart.

The War with Germany

1914 had found Richet, at sixty-four, too old to serve in the French army. His five sons and two sons-in-law, however, in his words, "performed their cruel duty." George and Gabriel Le Ber became interpreters for the British army while Charles was assigned duty as an ambulance doctor as his father had been in the Franco-Prussian war. Jacques served as sergeant in an infantry regiment and Albert taught at an aeronautical school for a time but left to become a fighter pilot. Son-in-law Edmond Lesné directed four military hospitals with very little help and Alfred, the youngest son served in the infantry. Louise and Adèle nursed patients with typhoid fever and Jeanne worked in a triage center for wounded soldiers. The other girls were in late stages of pregnancy.

Recalling the Start of the Tragedy

In 1918 Richet wrote to his children with these thoughts and recollections:[2]

This atrocious, monstrous war, a thousand-fold absurd, has in four years changed my whole life. I will try to describe it all to my dear children, writing my recollections of those days of cruel hardship in a simple straightforward way. I will omit empty phrases and simply describe the course of my thoughts, my deep emotions and perhaps some possibly useful things that I did. I am writing without notes in the chance of inspiration. Here am I, open and frank on a beautiful day in November 1918, my spirit crushed with grief by the death of my [son] dear Albert, my hero! I am in a rustic château, its roof destroyed by bombs and carpenters and German prisoners around me noisily working on the walls. There is a stool, a stove that rages (almost as furiously as I do), windows covered with paper, a cot . . . what does it matter? I must find out whether an infusion of horse plasma can save the lives of the wounded, our poor heroic wounded, who have lost their own blood.

During the final days of July, 1914, I was at the Ile Ribaud with my faithful [boatman] Joseph. I had two concerns, my *Histoire Universelle* . . . I had corrected the final proof. Mr. Berger in Berlin had started the [German] translation. My other concern was with the supply of zomine. I had a contract with Guilbaud and Grigaut in Antwerp that yielded me a 15 percent royalty but there was a clause that provided for cancellation within six months if the work had not begun. I went fishing, had a very good catch and then went to work on my book, *Pensées de Joachim Legris*. I was much affected and uneasy about the political news in the papers. The infamous ultimatum of the Austrians to Serbia, the vile aggression of Austria against Belgrade, the willingness of [Kaiser] Wilhelm to leave the Austrians free to commit this new rape! It all upset me greatly as did especially the state of mind of the newspapers. They were outrageously chauvinistic saying that we must not abandon Russia. I also happened to know that Poincaré with the sinister D. [Doubtless Ambassador to Russia, Delcassé] was preparing an offensive alliance against Germany. Happily, I have faith in [the newly elected Premier René] Viviani. I felt that to make war, a more terrible war than we have ever seen, for a few Serbian bandits would not be very interesting. The life of a French citizen is worth the life and honor of 50 Serbs. I believed in the good sense of the public. I was optimistic, but upon seeing what happened and what is happening now I believe only in the immense ineptitude of the people.

Saturday I left for Port Gros at five in the morning, greatly tormented. I returned with an enormous marlin weighing ten kilograms which I planned to take to my friend Guidon-Lesour later in the day. Noting that the gunners of the fleet off the coast of the Île d'Hyère were engaging in target practice as usual, I was fully reassured. It is not possible that one would amuse himself shooting if there were a declaration of war. Sunday morning the 1st of August, a day to remember forever: I left for Port Gros at half past 4 a.m. (to pick up my fishing boat *Circé* for another day of angling). When I arrived, what a surprise to see an old steamboat with an officer and soldiers of the Corps of Engineers. They had come to remove all of the pitiful armaments remaining at Port Gros. The adjutant told me that war had been declared at 4 o'clock the previous afternoon. It was a thunderbolt. I had to return to Paris immediately. Without delay I left, but the moment the *Circé* was unmoored someone came running and shouting, "take me and my wife." It was the very pleasant young Thomasset, almost a child. There were not forty years between him and his wife together. "I will be glad to take you" I said, "but I warn you that this won't be a pleasure trip. Whether or not you get seasick I will take you to Marseille and under no conditions will we change our course." It was 7:30 in the morning when I arrived at Île Ribaud. I told Elodie that she must leave with me and return to Paris with only a half an hour to pack. Girard [the caretaker] and his wife cried when we left. Poor Île Ribaud that I adored and still adore. I haven't seen it since that fatal day.

There were [the boatmen] Joseph and Théophile—who had been wounded and lost an eye—during the war (1870), Elodie, Théophile's wife and Thomasset and his wife. I decided not to go to Toulon because I thought the harbor would be too crowded. Since the sea was relatively calm with fairly strong swell and little wind, I decided to sail to Marseille. As we passed by Toulon at a distance of 3 km a large torpedo boat bore down on us and from it came a shout telling us to raise the flag. "No," I replied, "because it would call attention to us." The torpedo boat then quickly passed, turned and stopped in front of us. After we had identified ourselves they let us go on. The sea got rougher. Thomasset and his wife had collapsed at the rear of the boat, weak and silent. They were poor and didn't know how they would be able to manage away from le Ribaud. Then the tiller broke but we were able to steer anyway. At 3 P.M. we arrived at Marseille. *Circé* had performed wonderfully. Joseph and Théophile had been called to duty and here I was in Marseille. There was unbelievable noise and confusion at the railroad station. I went to see Mme. Livon. She was amazed when I declared the criminal folly of war. I began to understand human stupidity. I dined with Elodie and Mme. Charles Livon at the Hotel Terminus in Marseille. There was no room in the train but I learned that there was one car reserved for members of the legislature that were heading to Paris for a meeting. Although I had forgotten their names I asked them to let me ride with them. They were quite agreeable and there I was riding to Paris like a legislator. We were able to pass Elodie off as a nurse since she had somehow picked up an identifying arm band. I lost Thomasset and his wife in the station. The trip [to Paris] was lengthy, desperately long.

The next morning at 6 o'clock we arrived at Dijon where there were innumerable soldiers. I saw three or four battalions being swallowed up in the stairway leading beneath the quay. It was as if they were marching down to their doom! These poor children, (they were only children). They were neither sad nor joyous, neither singing nor weeping. They were driven by the fatalistic resolve: "Since we must go, let us go." Well, when one is young and vigorous one is attracted to the unknown with great adventurous emotions. No, they were not sad. How many more such children are there like those children carrying knapsacks and filing down the station steps, busy and bewildered, each trying to stick close to his company. Of the 6000 soldiers that left Dijon, perhaps 600 are alive and well today.As our train continued more news arrived. In the stations, there was excitement among hordes of young women, standing close to their men and carrying small bundles and weeping. We passed houses along the way where we saw women and their children standing waving to the train and wishing bon voyage. On Tuesday morning at Sens we were joined in our compartment by the mayor, M. Corret, also a senator who had bad news that Germany had overrun Belgium. We also learned that Britain had joined our side. That news gave me a clear and thoroughly confident conviction that with Britain on our side we could not be vanquished. France and Britain united are invincible, a conviction that turned out to be true. Germany's invasion of Belgium was a *colossal* error. Their declaration of war was a crime. The submarine war was a crime and an error. The combination of three (*sic*) crimes and three errors brought Germany's downfall. Finally by Tuesday afternoon we had arrived in Paris. I saw my dear wife who was awaiting me impatiently. That evening our five sons and two sons-in-law, Gabriel and Edmond dined with us. All seven and their wives were full of fervor and confidence.

The month that followed was frightful. News arrived rarely and what did come was disastrous. We could only get the truth through bribery. We were stupefied to learn that the Germans had arrived at the river Somme. How is it possible that they have penetrated so far! At first there was great enthusiasm for the Belgians. Everyone was speaking about their admirable resistance at Liège. Many of those whom I saw had a real fervor for the war. The newspapers in their blind nationalistic fury engaged in jingoistic rhetoric which disheartened me. One day I met a medical writer on the rue Jacob who said to me: "You were once a pacifist but I forgive you." "I have no need of your forgiveness," I replied, "You don't know to whom you are speaking." He offered me his hand but I refused it. I have recounted that incident in verse in *La Paix par le droit*. Finally, during the last days of August, after the capture of Maubeuge and the fall of Charleroi, the lightening speed of the German advance that now menaced Paris convinced my wife to leave Paris for Conqueiranne with Alfred, Adèle, Jeanne, Valérie, and the children. She went but not without great difficulty. The trains were jammed with people. At the same time the government, fearing the arrival of the Germans in Paris, retreated to Bordeaux. Although there was no one in the government offices to give me an official mandate, I decided to take off for Italy, where I had many friends, in an effort to persuade Italy to join France against the Germans. Not wishing to make the trip alone I asked my good friend André Weiss to accompany me. He agreed. The substitution of safe conduct passes for passports hadn't been enacted as yet so we had no difficulty leaving but my poor unlucky laboratory assistant, Jean, who was later killed in the war, had to spend the entire night in the station in order to save us two seats. The previous evening I had told Landouzy of my plan. He listened but made no reply except to shake his head.

The next morning at 7 he came into my room while I was still in bed. His manner was grave and, following a custom that he had adopted in time of war, he wore the insignia of a Commanduer de la Légion d'Honneur around his neck. He closed my opened window and said: "You don't think your departure is hazardous, it is very serious, no, it is impossible." He added with tears in his voice, "The Prussians will be here in three days. They will know in advance that you have gone to Italy to make propaganda against them. Since you have no family here and there is no one here but me, they will punish me for you and then go about pillaging the house. You can't leave!" Despite the gravity of the moment I had an impulse to laugh, but I did not do so. I contented myself with my usual custom and responded gently: "I will think it over."

The following day Weiss and I left for Chambéry, Modane, and Turin. What a spectacle to see Paris, like a desert, not illuminated and the madness at the station! I have never seen such a sight, even in the most tragic hours. Along the way we picked up groups of people who were fleeing the invasion. What a trip! The town of Meaux had been evacuated. The Germans had arrived at the gates of Paris! I could see Paris delivered up in flames and destroyed, perhaps it was to be an unavoidable defeat with my sons, my brave sons thrown into the furnace. What will become of them? What will be their fate? What will become of France? We stopped for a few hours in Dijon. My son Albert was on leave. He had left his antiaircraft company to enter pilot school because he said: "Antiaircraft batteries are simply a form of ambush." I saw how much in love he and his young wife were. They had only been married a few months. He had rented a little peasant's cottage at Vic Sur Ouche. I have a tender memory of having breakfast there in an orchard among the trees. How happy they were to be together! What joy I had to find them there and give them news of all the family. After a few hours we left, Weiss and I, for Chambéry. We devoured the newspapers telling of the resistance at the Marne. The great battle of the Marne was the greatest of all ages . . . but it amounted only to a little patch of blue among the dark clouds of defeat.

Richet and Weiss were welcomed in Italy and felt that their words had had some influence. At Bologna Richet was enthusiastically received by a large audience of students and faculty from the university. Although he spoke in French with an interpreter, they seemed to understand his words and afterwards the students stormed the Austrian Consulate, shouting and breaking windows. He was also well received in Ferrara, Milan, Venice, Genoa, and Florence. Whether or not because of their efforts, Italy soon joined the war on the side of the Allies. Richet then tried to carry out a similar mission to Romania but was rebuffed by the government of that country. Thereafter he traveled to Russia, Sweden, Norway, and Great Britain pleading France's cause in the war.

While telling of the visit to Italy with Weiss, Richet included a lengthy account of "the beautiful Countess Eleanore de Cossato" who entertained them at her palazzo. "I had the opportunity of meeting her," he wrote, "because she was a relative of Schrenk-Notzing." He added. "I don't deny that I was charmed by her beauty and vivacity." She recounted to him her sad early life and her childhood dreams. In response, Richet composed and recited a poem about her on the spot: the words roughly translated were

> She was earnest and sweet
> Dreaming along the byway
> With gentle dew on the moss
> Beneath her little feet.

He also described sightseeing trips with the countess by horse drawn carriage around Rome and other Italian cities. "I don't hesitate to say," wrote Richet, "that I was under the spell of her beauty and her disposition. The only town in Italy where we were not well received was Turin. The clerics were mobilized to oppose me. Nevertheless I spoke for three quarters of an hour before that hostile audience."

Work on Military Technology

After returning home from his European travels Richet went to visit the Institut Marey, Paul Bert's old laboratory in the Bois de Boulogne. After Paul Bert's death in 1886 and Marey's in 1904 Richet was given charge of supervising the direction of the institute. He found his student, Lucien Bull, at work there devising a way to track the trajectory of an enemy shell in order to precisely locate its source. The idea was to time the arrival of the noise of the cannon at three telephones set at a distance from one another and to calculate the trajectory from the delay in the sound reaching each phone. From the intersection of the parabolas one could identify the site of the cannon. Richet sought the help of the physicist and fellow Nobel laureate Gabriel Lippman who adapted the idea to a workable system. Bull, who as a protégé of Marey, had become known as a technical genius, refined the system further by connecting the impulse from the sound to a string galvanometer the movement of which was photographed to provide a graphic record in a fashion similar to early electrocardiograms. These artillery detectors were mounted in British Signal Corps vehicles.

Richet then collaborated with a man named de Roland to develop a device capable of detecting traces of the poison gas chlorine in the air. They found that minute amounts of chlorine would alter the resistance of a fine platinum wire. Working with another man named Sacerdote he then devised an even simpler chemical method using a glass vessel filled with potassium iodide. Contact with chlorine would release a visible iodine vapor that would stain a paper held over it.

A very brilliant wartime invention of Richet's was a highly practical combination between a life vest and a wet suit that protected the wearer against cold as well as against drowning. He designed a rubber garment lined with kapok that sheathed the entire body below the head. The feet were equipped with weights for balance and to permit the wearer to remain upright with his head out of the water. The suit was tested successfully in the lake in the Bois de Boulogne. Although the war was nearly over by the time the suit could be produced and no longer were sailors whose ships had been torpedoed plunged into the icy Atlantic ocean, Richet conceived civilian uses by bridge builders and others who had to work partially immersed in cold water.

The First War Casualties in the Family

While devoting much of his time and effort to developing useful machinery for the war Richet was also having to deal with catastrophes in his own family. His son-in-law Gabriel Le Ber, the husband of his daughter, Adèle, was killed at Verdun in 1916. Shortly thereafter Marthe, the pregnant wife of Charles fils, gave birth to a boy whom she named

Gabriel after her slain brother-in-law. Jacques was wounded in September at Reims and was taken prisoner. It was months before word of him reached home.

Richet responded to these tragedies in his characteristic manner, by getting involved, by speaking out. While the war was still raging he published an indictment of the promoters of the war, *Les Coupables*.[R 561] He identified as predominantly responsible the two emperors, Franz Joseph of Austria and Wilhelm II of Germany. "Wilhelm," he wrote, "resembled Napoleon in his determination to dominate the world." Richet found the diplomats to be also culpable as well as the German army with its Prussian military tradition. He also blamed the German press, declaring, "The press always supports the government in time of trouble." The socialists too were criticized for carping at the Austrians and their crown prince. Finally blame was extended to the neutral countries for doing nothing to stop aggressors. At the end, perhaps anticipating war crimes trials, he proposed that a means be found to punish the culpable aggressors.

Medical Service in the Combat Area

By now Richet wanted to involve himself more directly in the saving of lives and relief of suffering. He obtained permission to treat tuberculous soldiers hospitalized at Côte St. André with his beef juice concoction. He visited the trenches, the first aid stations and the field hospitals. These experiences prompted him to write a short book on procedures for nursing the wounding, *War Nursing: What Every Woman Should Know*.[R 589] Intended to serve as a guide to the care of soldiers, it covered such general topics as antisepsis, analgesia, and the management of shock. The book also emphasized the character qualities required in nurses, "devotion, docility, and activity."

He also served at the front near Vaux Varennes, Jonchery et Vasseny where he administered zomine mixed with champagne to wounded soldiers who were not in severe shock. According to Richet, "It seemed to help." For operative procedures he urged the use of chloralose in anesthesia. It proved useful but because it caused enhancement of bronchial mucus secretion chloralose could not be used for prolonged procedures in the most severely wounded. On the favorable side, and a boon to those patients suffering from traumatic shock, was the fact that under chloralose anesthesia not only was arterial pressure maintained but even increased. Richet calculated the depth of shock in the wounded from the ratio of urea nitrogen to total nitrogen in the urine. A low ratio indicated a poor prognosis since, in severe shock, the liver is unable to synthesize the nitrogen containing waste product, urea.

Plasma Transfusion

In the spring of 1918, Richet had an opportunity to try out other ideas for the treatment of wounded soldiers in shock. He knew of the transitory benefits of physiological saline in replacing blood lost. In addition, he had had some experience with blood transfusion, often catastrophic since, although blood types had already been discovered, the methods for testing them had not been developed for general use at the time. Several years earlier Richet had tried transfusing milk to replace blood volume.[R 20] The scheme had proved unsuccessful,[R 573] as had his experiments with various artificial solutions. He then tried blood plasma and found it more effective in the prevention of hemorrhagic shock in dogs. Now, in the war zone near Ockiney, he went into the trenches to treat wounded soldiers as promptly as possible with plasma from the blood of horses obtained by bleeding the animals into three-liter sterilized bottles containing nine grams of sodium citrate. After allowing the cells to settle, the plasma was decanted and injected intravenously. The first three soldiers so treated seemed to do well at first but later on died of septicemia. The war ended before Richet could experiment further with his plasma therapy. For his patriotism, dedication, and courageous service at the front, Richet was awarded the Croix de Guèrre.

The Loss of a Son

Shortly before the end of the war Richet's son Albert, a lieutenant pilot in Escadrille 117, was shot down accidentally by a French plane and killed, leaving his wife with three small daughters. He had won the cross of the Légion d'Honneur and eight citations. A few weeks before his death he had been wounded in the arm. At that time the minister of aviation M. Dumény offered him a post as director of a bombardment school. Breguet Aviation also offered him a promotion from his old job. He turned them both down and returned to combat. He was shot down at

Ainzy Le Château and was buried there. The reports that came to Richet were confusing at first. There seemed to be some hope that, although shot down, he might have survived. After frantic but futile efforts to obtain the facts from the military officials in Paris, Richet, Alfred's young wife and Adèle gathered at Carqueiranne. "We waited there in a state of anguish mingled with hope," wrote Richet. When the truth was finally evident he was bitter: "The French aviator who shot him down was afraid. The coward spent his ammunition at random in order to get back to his base as quickly as possible. . . . If I were God I might have pardoned him because there was no moral iniquity! But I am not God! I am not even a judge! I am only a poor man the death of whose courageous, noble, and intrepid son has plunged him into irreparable grief and I don't pardon him, I never will."

After the defeat of Germany and the Armistice in 1918 Richet, as much a patriot as a pacifist, pursued all the more vigorously his efforts to abolish war. He urged the elimination of armaments because, as he said, "without arms merchants there is no war." Concluding the account of his family's experiences in World War I Richet wrote, "Now Europe has been freed . . . millions are dead and 500 million are left in despair. They say that this will be the last war. In fifty to hundred years we will have another great war more terrible than this."

Passing the Torch to his Namesake

Richet's grim prediction was realized in only twenty-two years when his son Charles was carrying on the tradition of academic medicine and research, patriotism and pacifism. During the Second World War Charles *fils*, too old to serve in the army, was active in the Resistance and sheltered Allied pilots who were shot down over France. Eventually he was caught by the Germans who imprisoned him in Paris for seven months and then transferred him to Buchenwald for the remaining sixteen months of the war. Upon his liberation from the concentration camp he wrote to General de Gaulle urging him to make sure that German prisoners were properly treated according to the Geneva Convention.

Charles *fils* was appointed professor of nutrition in the Faculté de Médecine after the war. In his first lecture to the students he mentioned that seven members of the Faculté had been imprisoned in concentration camps and that only he among that group had survived. He kept in touch with as many of his fellow survivors of Buchenwald as he could find. He found among them an extraordinarily high prevalence of cancer. He himself suffered a cancer of the larynx which was surgically removed, requiring him to learn esophageal speech. In 1957 he published a monograph, *La pathologie de misère* (Richet *fils* 1957). It dwelt on what he felt were the consequences of life in the concentration camps and other experiences of human deprivation and degradation.

Richet's Post–World War I Adjustment

In the aftermath of World War I the depleted French economy, together with unusual family financial obligations, had considerably restricted the personal freedom that Richet had so highly prized throughout his life. Following the armistice Richet returned to his other missions, especially his effort to persuade the scientific establishment in France to take seriously and study systematically what he considered well-documented psychic phenomena. In 1923 Richet brought a copy of his just published *Traité de Métapsychique*[R 654] to a meeting of the Académie des Sciences and placed it on the table in the front of the lecture hall with these words: "To me it appears that the innumerable facts observed and recorded by such men as [Sir] William Crookes, Frederic Myers and many other widely respected scientists merit attention and should not be allowed to be annihilated by sarcasm or disdainful silence. I, too, bring to you my experimental contribution."

The book was widely reviewed because of Richet's prestige but nearly all of the reviewers complained about the quality of his evidence. Pierre Janet's review was sympathetic but critical of Richet's use of the testimony of other scientists as evidence (Janet 1923). The psychologist Henri Piéron wrote one of the gentlest reviews attributing Richet's lack of critique to his "genius," pointing out that he was good at hypothesis but weak on experimental rigor (Piéron 1922). Then Piéron with Georges Dumas (1866–1946) and the physiologist Louis Lapicque (1866–1952) set up a series of experiments in the physiology laboratory at the Faculté des Sciences in an attempt to replicate the materialization of ectoplasm which Richet had reported occurring at a séance with Eva C. (Marthe Béraud). No ectoplasm was produced. Nevertheless, during his final few years as professor, Richet continued his staunch advocacy of metapsychology. He was able to enlist very little support in France, however, and instead turned to his friends in Great Britain and the United States where there were active research societies.

In 1921 he returned to more conventional physiology and published with his son Charles a two-volume work called *Traité de Physiologie Medico-chirurgicale*, conceived as a companion piece to his father Alfred's famous book on *Surgical Anatomy*. A highly practical textbook, it emphasized the pertinence of knowledge of physiology to the treatment of disease, perhaps anticipating the style of Best and Taylor's *Physiological Basis of Medical Practice* (Brobeck 1973). The book was well received, so much so among surgeons that it became their standard authority on anesthesia and the hazard of cardiac arrhythmias due to oxygen deprivation of the brain. *Le Savant* appeared two years later, as did "L'Oeuvre de Pasteur." Richet also continued to publish work from his laboratory and did a bit of research, having become intrigued with learning the function of the spleen. He found that removal of the spleen from a dog did not compromise its survival, but noted that the dog required twice the usual amount of food to maintain its weight.

In his final lecture to the students he summarized the activities and achievements of his laboratory from 1881 to 1925.[R 667] He spoke of his discovery of the thermoregulatory functions of panting and shivering in dogs as his most significant contribution. The others he ranked in the following order: serotherapy (the discovery of passive immunity), zomotherapy (the beef juice treatment of tuberculosis and cancer), the development of resistance to poisonous metal salts by bacteria, and lastly anaphylaxis, the importance of which he felt had been "a bit exaggerated." He went on to acknowledge the help of collaborators, of instrument makers, others who created opportunities for him, and luck. He added a short homily and concluded, "what really mattered was my confidence in the invincible power of science."

Notes

1. The meaning of the literal translation of these words is a bit abstruse but the message is "to combine our voices (contributions to the world) would bring the richest reward."
2. I have translated this passage from Richet's *Mémoires* nearly verbatim except for correcting punctuation and omitting a few lines and parts of sentences, such as minor asides that had no bearing on the narrative and often impaired the clarity of the meaning.

8

The Final Decade 1925–1935

After retiring as professor, Richet began to apply much of his energy to what others called spiritualism and the occult. In fact, he had intended that his final lecture to the students be dedicated to metapsychology (métapsychique) but, at the dean's request, he agreed to devote it to a review of the work of his laboratory from 1881 to 1925, emphasizing its place in the history of physiology.[R 666] Metapsychology then became the topic of his next to last lecture. He began it as follows: "Before leaving this chair that I have held for so long, I would like to acquaint you with the outlines of a new science, metapsychology, which is not yet part of the official teaching of physiology. Nevertheless, it constitutes an integral part of physiology and in the future, perhaps, it will be identified with classical physiology." Richet went on to declare that mind cannot be independent of matter, but rather is subject to its laws. Rejecting any notion of the supernatural, Richet contended that extrasensory perception implied a sixth sense, not yet studied. He declared that the ability of mediums to move unattached objects must depend on physiological mechanisms only rarely brought into play and still to be identified. His concluding words were "I imagine that one of the great tasks of the 20th century will be to give medical psychology its full range of development, but it is a great task for physiology to make it beautiful."[R 666]

Richet's publications after 1925 included twenty-five on the subject of metapsychology, most of which appeared in the *Revue Metapsychique*.

In 1928 he wrote *Notre Sixième Sens* which was promptly translated into English.[R 697] It contained a collection of more or less documented instances of clairvoyance that he had experienced or observed. He dedicated the book to a distinguished philosopher and colleague as follows: "This book of audacious physiology is dedicated to my eminent friend, Henri Bergson, the most profound thinker of modern times." In it he acknowledged a prior 1927 publication with the same title, but on a different subject, by Joseph Sinel.[R 697] Richet's ideas on metapsychology were treated publicly among scientists with forbearance because of his social and scientific standing, but, despite their appeal to several well-known intellectuals in France and elsewhere, privately they were ridiculed. Many of his former colleagues, and even members of his family took an apologetic attitude toward them. Some attributed his consorting with spiritualists to aberrations of an aging brain; this explanation, of course, did not apply in view of Richet's nearly lifelong interest in "strange" phenomena, and of his having even devoted his first publication in a scientific journal to his experiences with somnambulism.

After his retirement as professor, that side of Richet that loved solitude and contemplation came in for greater play as he grew older. He spent much of his time near the sea, thinking, writing and especially fishing. He built a device that measured ocean currents at Le Havre and made use of special instruments to locate fish.

Another Festschrift

In 1926, the year following Richet's retirement, the Académie de Médecine organized a second jubilee to honor Richet for his nearly forty years as professor (Loir 1926). The distinguished physicist and engineer, Paul Painlevé (1863-1933) who was prime minister of France at the time, presided over the meeting. One part of the occasion was devoted to expressions of congratulations and homage from former pupils andassociates,representatives of scientific societies in France and from twelve other nations. Another part of the program was devoted to presentations, mainly scientific, by distinguished scientists in Europe, Great Britain and North and South America. Appendix 8.1 lists the speakers and their topics. Prime Minister Painlevé commented on Richet's contributions to aircraft design, "whether it concerns ideas or experiments, spiritual aspirations or material progress, Richet has always been in the forefront. Recently when heavier than air transportation seemed impossible, it was not surprising that Charles Richet tried to achieve it." Painlevé then mentioned those whose feats of design and engineering had made aviation possible, beginning with Sir George Cayley (1773-1857) whom he credited with producing the first rational design of a flying machine in the early eighteenth-century. He added that the first plane that actually flew, made by Alphonse Penaud (1850-1880) in 1871, was powered by rubber bands. A decade later came the experiments of Victor Tatin who was soon to be joined by Charles Richet. Finally, Painlevé referred to Richet's development of the helicopter with Louis and Jacques Breguet in 1907.

Among the most interesting presentations at the meeting was one by Graham Lusk (1866–1932) on the specific dynamic action of food. In it he cited the contributions of Richet, mentioning him in sequence between Rubner and DuBois, but he did not credit Richet with any notable discovery in the food-fuel area. Sir Charles Sherrington wrote about summation and recruitment in reflex muscular contraction and inhibition, emphasizing that summation is not only a feature of neural excitation but of inhibition as well. He identified Richet's early work with the crayfish as a "classical contribution." Prof. Auguste Pi-Suñer of the Faculty of Medicine at Barcelona, Spain pointed out the unifying theme of Richet's investigations of seemingly scattered topics in physiology. To illustrate he chose three publications, *Les réflexes psychiques*,[R 226] *La défense de l'organisme*[R 372] and Richet's presentation at the Congress of Physiology in Vienna in 1910, *L'humorisme ancien et l'humorisme moderne*.[R 509] "These, together with others of Richet's work," said Pi-Suñer, "contain innovative ideas and perceptions in physiology and psychology." He declared that Richet had modernized the concept of reflex function, dispelling the earlier notion of Marshall Hall (1790–1857), the British physician-scientist who was one of the first to recognize and study reflexes (Hall 1833). Hall had declared that reflexes and voluntary actions involved totally separate mechanisms. Richet, building on the more recent work of Ivan Mikhailovich Sechenov (1829–1905) (Sechenov 1952), considered automatic behavior, as in reflexes, and behavior in response to will or emotions to be at opposite ends of a continuum of increasing complexity of nervous connections. According to Pi-Suñer, Richet's research was unified by a concept of defense of the organism through an integrated system of neural regulatory mechanisms.

Ivan Pavlov reported his observations on temperamental differences in dogs. He showed that the patterns of neurosis differ from one breed to another. He also reported producing neurosis in dogs by persistent attempts to reestablish a conditional reflex after a two-month interruption of the experiments.

Walter Cannon's paper was particularly notable because it outlined clearly for the first time his theory of homeostasis, the normal maintenance of constituents of the blood and body fluids at an approximately constant concentration. As mentioned earlier, in his presentation he acknowledged his indebtedness to Richet's work. Cannon began his talk with a quote from Richet's article "Functions of Defense" in his *Dictionnaire de Physiologie*, volume 4 published in 1900.[R 419], "The living being is stable. It must be so in order not to be destroyed, dissolved or disintegrated by the colossal forces, often adverse, which surround it. In a sense it is stable because it is modifiable—the slight instability is the necessary condition for the true stability of the organism." He also included a quotation from Claude Bernard to whom, of course, both he and Richet were indebted.

Paul Portier, who had been Richet's collaborator in the original work on anaphylaxis without seeming to have maintained much interest in it, described experiments that showed the antennae of butterflies to be essential to the maintenance of equilibrium during flight.

Richet's son, Charles, spoke on individual variations among organisms of the same species, pointing out their importance, especially among humans. He argued that physiological norms tell less about a species than do its individual differences. "Clearly, among humans," he declared, "it is the deviations from the norm that have defined the capacity of the species."

Louis Lapicque professor of general physiology at the Sorbonne, provided an interesting reflection on what he considered to be the fundamental physiological mechanisms involved in poetry. He pointed out that while some people experience poetry as an intellectual exercise, others see it as an exercise in sensuality. "Good poetry," said Lapicque, "offers both." To understand poetry requires on the one hand, concentrated reasoning with all distractions shut out. In physiological terms such a sharp focus of attention involves inhibition of some sensory pathways. On the other hand the music and imagery of poetry call for a breadth of sensitivity and openness to stimuli of all sorts, thus requiring activation of widespread sensory circuits. Poetry, then, provides an experience in sensuality as well as in cognitive abstraction. According to Lapicque, when either the intellectual or the sensual element gets out of hand, poetry is inferior, as is music that lacks the proper balance of intellectual discipline and feeling. Finally, with a characteristically Gallic touch he added, "the possession of a woman amounts to very little when compared to the infinitely complex involvement of the nervous system in what we call love." He reminded the audience that Richet's most acclaimed writings were his poetry, the fables, *Pour les Grands et les Petits* and the poem for which he won the prize from the Académie Française, *La Gloire de Pasteur*. His plays, *Circé* and *Soeur Marthe* were also written in verse.

William Stirling (1851–1932) professor of physiology and dean of the Faculty of Medicine at Victoria University of Manchester, in a tribute to Richet's contributions to the history of medicine, discussed the historical introduction to his translation of Harvey's work. Stirling also praised Richet for his writings on Servetus and added further historical data from his own research. Maurice Arthus, who wrote the first important paper on immunology following Richet's explanation of anaphylaxis, elected to moralize about scientific research by propounding what he called the seven cardinal virtues of the experimenter. (1) scientific curiosity; (2) decisiveness; (3) mental flexibility; (4) a critical sense; (5) precision; (6) love of order; and (7) self control. Arthus did not connect Richet with any part of this litany of perfection.

Arthus' presentation borrowed heavily from the preface of his major publication, *De l'Anaphylaxie à Immunité*, (Arthus 1921) intended as a guide for young physiologists or those contemplating a career in physiology. The book reflected Arthus' single minded approach to science and his rigidly disciplined mode of inquiry which contrasted sharply with that of Richet whose energy of inquiry propelled him into several areas of study (Longcope 1943). Although Arthus' research was inspired by Richet's discovery of anaphylaxis, the very breadth and extent of Richet's endeavor may explain Maurice Arthus' failure to identify Richet with the seven cardinal virtues of a scientist. According to Henry E. Sigerist (1891–1957) Johns Hopkins' professor of the history of medicine, who prepared the English translation of Arthus' preface to his book *De l'Anaphylaxie à l'immunité*, Arthus' view of physiology was vastly different from that of Richet and was somewhat closer to Richet's prescription for a scientist in his book *Le Savant*.[R 649] Sigerist quoted a statement made by Arthus in 1920 that was clearly at odds with Richet's view: "Strongly impressed by great results obtained, some people have thought that all manifestations of life, even the most immaterial, should belong to the realm of physiology. We believe this to be a mistake and think that it is important to separate clearly the material or physiological facts from the immaterial or psychological ones" (Sigerist 1943).

Arthus' homilies by no means put Richet beyond the pale. It was not unusual for prominent medical scientists to invest themselves seriously in activities outside of their main endeavor. Rudolph Virchow was highly respected as an anthropologist and archaeologist who, with Heinrich Schliemann (1822–1890), made excavations at the presumed site of ancient Troy. Richet shared with Virchow his broad view of the science of man as representing the whole range of human endeavor and experience. For the most part Richet seems to have reconciled his own intellectual peregrinations with his broad view of physiology and his obligations toward mankind.

At the end of the jubilee when all of the speakers had been heard, Maréchal Foch came forward to decorate Richet with the insignia of a Grand Officier de la Légion d'Honneur for valorous service to his country. The presence of Maréchal Foch, as well as President Paul Painlevé's recognition of Richet's remarkable insight into aircraft design, Stirling's tribute to his scholarly accomplishments, and Lapicque's praise of his poetry indicated a regard for Richet that clearly transcended his significance as a physiologist. The occasion was one to celebrate a great humanist, a model of broad cultivation and creativity, a civilizing influence in society.

Philosophical Views and Publications

Among the intellectual forebears of Charles Richet might be included Paracelsus (1493–1541), who early expressed the broad vision of clinical medicine held by Richet, recognizing especially the importance of chemistry. Paracelsus (1493–1541) wrote in his *De Moto Pharmacandi*, "A physician must be a philosopher; that is to say he must dare to use his own reason and not cling to antiquated opinions and book authorities, he must above all be in possession of that faculty called intuition that cannot be acquired by blindly following the footsteps of another. He must be able to see his own way" (Paracelsus 1891). His commitment to not only seeing but pursuing his own way was Richet's closest resemblance to Paracelsus. There is even an intellectual propinquity between Paracelsus and Richet in their fascination with unfamiliar and mysterious forces such as animal magnetism. Indeed, Hartman credits Paracelsus with the discovery of animal magnetism, popularized in the eighteenth-century by Franz Anton Mesmer (1734–1815). Hartman, on page 227, quotes

Paracelsus, "Man possesses a magnetic power by which he may attract certain effluvia of a good or evil quality in the same manner as a magnet will attract particles of iron" (Hartman 1891). On page 231, Hartman states, "Lessing proved in 1769 that the real discoverer of animal magnetism was Paracelsus." On page 215 Hartman quotes some of Paracelsus' clinical wisdom: "the character of the physician may act more powerfully on the patient than all the drugs employed." On page 216, "the physical surroundings of the patient may have a great influence on the course of his disease. If he is waited upon by persons who are in sympathy with him, it will be far better for him than if his wife or his attendants wish for his death."

Richet held the materialistic view that thoughts and emotions are to be found in the physio-chemical machinery of the brain. Paracelsus, however, viewed the brain as an expressive *instrument* or *device*, not a *cause* of intellectual and emotional behavior. From his *De Veribus Morborum*, Hartman quotes, "wisdom and reason and thought are not contained in the brain but they belong to the invisible universal spirit which feels through the heart and thinks by means of the brain. All these powers are contained by the invisible universal and become manifest through material organs." On matters of identity of the spirit, Richet and Paracelsus also differed widely. Paracelsus stated that "the beginning of wisdom is the beginning of supernatural power" (Paracelsus 1891). Richet rejected the supernatural and looked forward to the day when all presumably supernatural events would be explained by the laws of physics and physiology.

Louis Pasteur, who more than any man served as a model for Charles Richet, did not share Richet's materialistic beliefs. As René Dubos tells it in his biography of Pasteur, "speaking in 1874 at the graduation exercises at the Collège d'Arbois, where he had been a student, he affirmed that religious convictions are founded on the impregnable rock of direct personal experience" (Dubos 1950). "The man of faith," Pasteur declared "believes in a supernatural revelation. If you tell me that this is incompatible with human reason I shall agree with you, but it is still more impossible to believe that reason has the power to deal with the problems of origins and ends." Dubos goes on to quote from Pasteur's remarks upon his induction into the Académie des Sciences: "The Greeks understood the mysterious power of the hidden side of things. They bequeathed to us one of the most beautiful words in our language—the word enthusiasm—En theos—an inner God." Dubos explained that Pasteur, at his election to l'Académie Française, argued with his opponent Ernest Renan that "pretending to explain human behavior in scientific terms fails to take into account the most important of all the positivist notions, that of infinity. Although an inescapable conclusion of human thinking, the notion of infinity is incomprehensible to human reason . . . more incompatible with it than are all the miracles of religion." Pasteur added, "I see everywhere in the world the inevitable expression of the concepts of infinity. It establishes in the depth of our hearts a belief in the supernatural." Whether or not Richet reflected on these words is not known. He surely must have read them.

Some of his friends doubted that Richet had remained unyielding in his views on what many would call the human spirit. His friend Eugene Osty (Osty 1936) quoted a paragraph from Richet's last monograph, *Au Secours*: "Little by little I have touched higher levels and have surveyed the beyond of the ordinary world which surrounds us."[R 738] Osty thought it indicated that Richet had abandoned the materialistic views expressed 40 years earlier in his *Essai de Psychologie-Générale*.[R 297] Oliver Lodge, on the other hand, believed that Richet's former convictions remained unshaken. "To the end of his life," Lodge wrote, "Richet in public remained an agnostic and a disbeliever in the spiritual explanation. In private, he has confessed to me that he was sometimes nearly bowled over by the evidence; but, on the whole, he adhered to his lifelong conviction of the materialistic aspect of the universe. His scientific reputation was thereby saved, and his experience was all the more valuable because it testified only to the bare facts which, although admittedly incredible from the scientific point of view, were not employed to bolster up any spiritualistic hypothesis. On those terms we agreed to differ, and yet remained close friends. He (Richet) lost a favorite son in the war but held no communication with him, though at times he was sorely tempted to do so" (Pierson 1940). Two years before his death Richet did hint at a belief in the afterlife.

Richet thus appears to have maintained his public posture, if not his conviction, about the hereafter until his death. According to his son, Alfred, however, he ultimately accepted the spiritual ministrations of Msgr. Baudrillart, rector of the Institut Catholique a few days before his death.

Philosophical Works

Most of Richet's philosophical works were published after he had
retired from the chair at the university in 1925. They fluctuated between
an almost cynical pessimism to high aspiration and hope for the future.
L'Homme Impuissant appeared in 1927.[R 686] In it he reviewed man's
physical limitations, "we are trapped by nature's laws," he wrote. He also
took a pessimistic view of the future of civilization, "the influence of
artists, writers, politicians, scientists, etc. is minuscule when seen quan-
titatively in terms of how many people in the world for generations pay
attention." He listed a few famous people—"people who have disciples
and whose work changes the course of the world, but they make up a
small percentage." He expressed contempt for the crude masses. "There
are vast numbers of them even in France, the most refined country in the
world. The masses are so enormous that the individual human is nothing.
What stupid things you hear everywhere—even in an elegant salon. For
an ambitious young author it is almost impossible to break through the
wall of obscurity."

Concerning man's intellectual limitations he wrote, "Man suffers
because he wants to know and can't—oysters don't suffer—the hoi polloi
don't suffer because they don't question—but there is joy in question-
ing." He then dwelt on man's moral limitations and his apparent inability
to deal generously with his fellow man, adding, "People know the
importance of cooperation but they are unable to cooperate because of
their jealousies, greed, hatred, etc. Liberté, Egalité, Fraternité, we have
none of these." To illustrate the proper attitude he quoted a saying of his
grandfather, "If someone's words hurt me, I am sad for the entire day.
When it is I who have said the hurtful words, I am sad for the entire
month." Toward the end of the book he offered this homily: "No one is
better or wiser than anyone else; be modest, almost humble."[R 686]

L'Homme Impuissant also contains some clouded predictions. In one
of the most unfortunate of these Richet wrote, "People used to concern
themselves with the effects that whale's tails exert on the waves of the
sea. Today they are concerned with amino acids. The theory of amino
acids does not appear to me to be destined for an important future." He
also made the emphatic prediction, already mentioned, that there can
never be flight into space. "We can see lights billions of miles away but
we can only approach 1.5 km toward them. Why have we such a piercing

view and such feeble muscles?" In another prediction he anticipated that there would be a 10 degree cooling of earth in a thousand years, and also that because of oxygen slowly leaking out of our atmosphere, eventually there would not be enough of it to support life.

Ironically thirty-nine years earlier in his first lecture as professor (*Leçon Inaugurale*), Richet had warned against predictions in science. After quoting several instances of an achievement having been predicted by scientists to be impossible he said: "Gentlemen, you may be assured that science has in store many such surprises. It is foolhardy ever to declare: 'Science cannot '"[R 271, 237]

L'Intelligence et l'homme was published in 1927. It is an exhortative essay on the proper rules for civilization.[R 687] He espoused a biological theory based on the laws of attraction (gravity) that provide for "growth, differentiation and efficiency of function." With acknowledgement to Count Leo Tolstoi (1828–1910) whose strong convictions about moral responsibility were well known, Richet took an almost religious position that the gradual development of life, intelligence, conscience and a sense of proper duty were part of the destiny of planet Earth.

In a 1930 publication, *L'age d'or et l'age de l'or* (The golden age and the age of money) he examines man's objectives, money, power, ease, self-indulgence, etc. and finds them invalid and counterproductive to world progress, peace and happiness. "Only through international communication, understanding and cooperation can these goals be achieved," he wrote, "A common language will be required [Richet favored Esperanto], without abandoning the traditional ones. More emphasis on science will be needed especially eugenics, the science of heredity to improve the human race."[R 711] In *La Grande Espérance* published in 1933, Richet is mainly concerned with a search for the purpose of life. "Why do you exist?" He asks in the first sentence. Then, enlarging on an argument in a paper he had written in 1884 called *L'Homme et l'intélligence* and shaping it according to what he perceived as Darwin's teachings, he declares, "Destiny equates with chance—the gamete determines everything."[R 145] He proposed human breeding, by law if necessary, toward further growth in human intelligence (which Richet equated with the soul) as generation after generation adds to the accumulation of knowledge and wisdom. "The ultimate purpose of man," he concludes, "is to have children and for children to increase in intelligence." Thus, perhaps, Richet anticipated the currently popular theory that the basic biological motive of individual animals, including man, is to perpetuate one's genes. He published in 1935 his final book, *Au Secours*, a call for help. In it he declares that he personally no longer needs help because he is near death, but he calls for help for: "noble ideas which are scorned by modern youth."

> Despite the clamors and sarcasms our old civilization appears superior to the pompous proclamations of the Germans, the bloody prejudices of the Soviets and the bizarre vases of the Chinese. Bring help to liberty, to truth, to science, to justice, to the sick, to peace, to metapsychology, to our Greco Roman civilization, Latin, Christian, French, devoted to progress. The west is menaced by the East. Bring help to our dear French language, to science, to dramatic arts, etc.[R 737]

Epilogue - Two Voices in a Dream

"This book was nearly finished," continued Richet,

> in fact I was correcting the page proofs while my thoughts strayed and a vague sleepiness crept over me. Was it a dream? I felt that I heard two voices distinctly calling my name but I wasn't afraid because I was in a state of believing that it was a dream. I demanded vigorously of the first voice: "who are you?" Then, after a long silence, the voice responded: "Your conscience; your life has differed greatly from your writings. You want to reform people but you don't realize that you must begin with yourself and must conform to the precepts which you preach." The voice fell silent and I felt myself overcome by a dark despair when suddenly another voice called me by name. With profound emotion I recognized the voice immediately, "Is it you", I asked, "my beloved grandfather?"

His grandfather consoled him, saying that by having tried, by having defended the truth, he had put in place a small stone in the immense edifice humanity will build for the future. The book concluded with the following statement:

> "I am the traveler who having arriving at the end of his voyage asks before an unknown portal whether or not he has followed the proper path."

The mention of the portal and his anxiety about whether or not he had "followed the proper path" evokes the recollection of Richet's promise to the Abbé Caron that he would study for the priesthood. This reverie in the twilight of his life contrasts with his sustained and forceful rejection of religion. His musing about the "portal" and the path also suggests a sense of regret over his failure to have held to a single-minded, "monastic" commitment to physiology as he had promised in his first lecture as professor. Only the sense that he had earned the approval of his grandfather lifted him from his melancholy. Richet had wanted desperately to have made a difference, to have left his mark. He had fully invested his talents and pursued his goals with energy and vitality but had moved in each of several directions a shorter distance than he might have had he pursued but one or two as had Pasteur, Bernard, Lippman, and Arthus.

A Final Presentation to the Académie de Sciences

In 1933, in his last address as president of the Académie des Sciences Richet's opening word were "Strike me, but first let me speak." He then reiterated his conviction that metapsychology should be taken seriously by scientists and should be studied as a branch of physiology.[R 727] He argued that as a new science, metapsychology was replacing the occult and supernatural metaphysics. He added that as a natural science, meta-psychology was still in a descriptive phenomenological stage that called for rigorous observation and careful recording of facts. He urged that it be nurtured so that eventually the underlying anatomical, physiological, and chemical components could be identified and the governing laws formulated. At this point Richet, within two years of the end of his life, and facing the skepticism and even scorn of his peers declared, "but I understand (science) in a far broader way than when I started. The science of life merges with a science of thought and I envision magnificent horizons in the future."[R 727]

In a commentary published shortly after Richet's death, Henri Bou-quet, who had been present at the Académie des Sciences and had heard the plea that metapsychology be taken seriously and studied scientifi-cally, wrote with admiration of his friend's courage and intellectual integrity (Bouquet 1935) on that occasion, Charles Richet, an aged man of undisputed distinction, presented his recently published book, *La Grande Espérance*[R729] to his colleagues. He was fully aware of the insults awaiting him. He knew that he would be treated as a fanatic if not as a fool, that some would even question his mental balance, that in any case he would be more scoffed at than taken seriously. Nevertheless he did what he considered his duty. Placing his book on the desk he said, "I request that I not be judged until I have been read. As rash as it may seem, this study had to be made and I had the courage to make it. The courage of a Savant is to declare what he believes to be true."

He was only repeating that day what, at age twenty, he had replied to his father who had reproached him for risking his future by his preoccupation with hypnotism: "one risks ones future by speaking the truth?" he asked. His future was not in peril either time. He had dared to speak out because he considered so-called occult or supernatural phenomena to be simply unfamiliar phenomena which should be studied just like any other puzzling observation. He parried his detractors with the comment "you are also the ones who denied the possibility of airplane flight!"

Richet had stood above the crowd not only in stature but in erudition, wealth and position. His attitude clearly matched his "nom de seigneur." referred to in the opening sentences of this book. Such pride and detachment probably contributed to his failure to attract the brightest students for his *foyer intellectuel* and to build a fully integrated laboratory program. Despite having to work almost alone following Portier's departure, Richet's study of anaphylaxis, triggered by his curiosity in the face of an unexpected and disappointing experimental result, established his extraordinary capability as a scientist. Had he persisted following his several other original observations and focused his efforts with single-minded determination in the almost monastic fashion for which he expressed such reverence in his *Le Savant*, would Charles Richet's name be accorded today a place of honor among medical scientists comparable to that of Pasteur or Bernard?

During the last year or two of his life Richet became increasingly frail. He found it difficult to get about but, according to Henri Bouquet, "he continued to come to the Institut (Académie des Sciences) because of his insatiable desire for knowledge; he listened with scrupulous attention to all of the presentations, even those on subjects unfamiliar to him . . . although his physical forces diminished rapidly, his brain remained fully capable" (Bouquet 1935). Apparently sensing the imminence of death, however, Richet gave the portrait of his father Alfred and also that of his mother Adèle, painted by Baudry, to his oldest son, George. At the time of his death three manuscripts were ready for publication, *L'Europe au XIXe siècle Les femmes immortelles* and *L'avenir de la science*.

On December 4, 1935 suffering from what was called a longstanding bronchopneumonia (more likely the pulmonary congestion of heart failure), Charles Richet died at home.

Louis Pasteur's grandson Pasteur Vallery-Radot wrote in an obituary published in *La Revue des Deux Mondes*, "Charles Richet astonished his

142 Brain, Mind, and Medicine

contemporaries by his intellectual audacity; his imagination was always aroused as was his enthusiasm about life . . . and his insatiable appetite for understanding."

Richet's wife Amélie lived on for nearly twenty years in their home at 15 rue de l'Université, keeping in close touch with the children and grandchildren. She even had an opportunity to see several great-grand-children before her death in 1954.

Appendix 8.1

THE PROGRAM OF RICHET'S 1926 FESTSCHRIFT

Notes

1. The last sentence of his book *La Grande Espérance* was "you bear all the painful responsibilities of life, you elevate yourself, and when death shall come you will be able to sleep (doubtless to reawaken) in all serenity."[R 729]
2. The union of the egg and the sperm.

9

Coda

Charles Richet valued all aspects of independence, academic independence and freedom from social restrictions, although in matters of social civility and the precise use of language he was a strict conformist. As his colleague Jean-Louis Faure (1863–1944) expressed it, "He was above all a free spirit. It is impossible to separate among the talents that contributed to his work, his quality as a scientist, a poet or a dreamer" (Faure 1935).

As a youth, Richet was financially independent and free to follow his inclinations. He did not appear to be strongly driven toward any particular career. Even his decision to marry was made when he had "neither a desire nor a distaste for marriage." Richet opted for a medical education "because I thought it would please my father." His decision to qualify for a science degree as well was made on an impulse when he and his friend, Henri Hermite happened to spot a notice that qualifying examinations were to be held. Later when Richet acquired the prestige and responsibilities of a savant, respectful as he was of the monastic virtues of his scientific models, Pasteur, Bernard and Lippmann, he seemed to identify more closely with the debonair qualities of his friend Antoine Breguet.

Richet's personality was in many ways contradictory. "The true Savant," wrote Richet, "is unencumbered by personal ambition, seeks no glory and is not jealous of his achievements."[R 649] Richet's prolonged resentment of von Behring's unwillingness to acknowledge his original work on serotherapy, however was at odds with his ideal. Even years later when his brother-in-law, Landouzy, wrote about serotherapy, failing to give Richet a prominent citation, Richet wrote in his *Mémoires*: "I assure you I was embittered, I was exasperated. My dear wife, who is wiser than I, managed to calm me." In another incident, Edouard Brissaud (1852–1909), a friend and faculty colleague, also failed to mention Richet in a lecture on serotherapy. Richet promptly sent him a letter breaking off their friendship. When the poor fellow came to him in tears to apologize, Richet forgave him and said, "there is no longer any cloud between us."

For his part Richet was usually meticulous about assigning credit where credit was due except when the glory of France was involved. He took pains to acknowledge his collaborators. On his manuscripts the names of authors were nearly always listed alphabetically. He seemed simply unable, however, to accept the nearly inevitable experience of a scientist to have others ignore his priority of discovery.Thus, on the one hand he extolled humility and selfless service and on the other he manifested a strong need for attention and recognition.

Further characterizing a savant, Richet wrote, "He should not be subject to distraction. His full time and energy should be devoted to his field of enquiry. He should not look for practical applications of his work. The interest of a research is not in practical application, a precept I consider so fundamental and essential that it dominates all others . . . If you would discover a new truth, do not seek to know what use will be made of it. Do not ask in what way medicine or commerce or industry may profit."[R 649] His own persistent efforts to find cures hardly reflected that conviction.

Although, as a medical scientist Richet was jealous of credit, vain and sensitive to slights, he was also generous and magnanimous with colleagues and even rivals. While convinced of his own superiority and that of the white race, he was also concerned about the human suffering throughout the world. Although a chauvinistic and patriotic Frenchman he worked to promote peace and freedom in other countries, notably Poland.[1] As a vocal champion of justice he wrote dozens of articles aimed at perfecting the human race, achieving world peace, and relieving human suffering. His dedication to such lofty goals was not as a religious believer but as what today might be called a liberal humanist. Richet, who held that physiology was the rational basis of clinical medicine, worked toward practical applications of his observations and discoveries. His dedication to unbiased science seemed to him quite compatible and coherent with his concern for the relief of human suffering. In his view, the task of the scientist was to ennoble and bring benefit to society. He considered his efforts on behalf of eugenics to be a part of this commitment.

So were his pacifism and his republican politics, so greatly influenced by his grandfather Renouard, all serious commitments, as was his long devotion to bibliography. Since physiology was still a relatively new science as distinct from anatomy, it was easy for him to justify his interest in gathering together in one series of volumes the existing relevant physiological literature.

Richet's pupil and later colleague, André Mayer analyzed the paradox of Richet's deep devotion to science and his susceptibility to distractions including not only his literary and bibliographic work but also his preoccupation with social causes (Mayer 1936). Mayer believed that Richet's basic goal was "to understand man from all angles, to involve himself with everything human." Mayer saw this as a response to the influences of the times as expressed in the writings of Destutt de Tracy and Condillac (discussed in chapter 2) that were "enormously popular with the youth of his time." Rather than focusing on isolated physical and chemical processes in human beings, Richet was attracted by the explanatory potential of Tracy's ideology through which aspects of human thought, emotion, individual behavior and social organization may be ultimately understood as a unified concept based on natural laws. According to Mayer, Richet believed that the proper path toward such understanding was that pursued by the naturalists of the eighteenth-century, including Baron George Cuvier (1769–1832) who coined the word "organism."[2] He felt that one must see mankind in an evolutionary perspective, extending over millions of years of adaptation. This view Richet defended in a letter published in 1902 in the *Revue Scientifique*.[R] [428] It led to an exchange of letters with the poet Sully-Prudhomme. Their discussion revolved around the concept of biological purpose, expressed as les causes finales, (the ultimate reason for life).[3] Mayer's explanation for Richet's remarkable success was that he understood the importance of what Jacques Loeb, a contemporary of Richet, called the study of the organism as a whole.[4] Thus, he pointed out, much of Richet's research was necessarily descriptive, phenomenological and less concerned with detail than with the biological significance of his observations. Exceptions were the step by step investigations of the properties of the muscles and nerves of the crayfish, his first research effort, and his discovery and clarification of anaphylaxis. "More often," wrote Mayer, "he seemed to approach a discovery of a series of leaps. First comes the sharp observation, followed by a quick grasp of its significance and then, skipping over details, comes a formulation in terms of a biological adaptation. He did not wish to allow extremes of detail to delay his work; there is still too much that is unknown" (Mayer 1936).

Mayer explained Richet's persistent concern with therapeutics as stemming from the clear medical application of the work of Pasteur who had "brought medicine and medical science together in an entirely new era, profoundly changing man's vulnerabilities and capabilities. Beyond this, Richet believed that the ultimate understanding of psychology and its control in the nervous system would free man from his obstinate self-destructiveness, and that selective breeding would raise him to a higher evolutionary level."

Apart from his recurrent tendency to look for practical applications of his work, Richet's mind was usually attracted to puzzles of any kind. In medical school subjects without puzzles, notably anatomy, failed to interest him. During anatomy classes, according to Marilisa Juri, "he consoled himself by writing verses and plays" (Juri 1965). Similarly, during his first internship under the surgeon, Lefort, not being attracted to the intellectual challenge of surgical practice, he focused his attention on patients who, after anesthesia, experienced hallucinations and personality changes. Richet experimented on these patients again and again with hypnotism. The phenomenon had intrigued him ever since his youthful experience of hypnotizing a friend of his younger sister.

The ultimate puzzle for Richet was the brain, the regulator of the human being in all respects, providing the mechanism for ideas, talents and emotions as well as ultimately controlling all bodily functions. In nearly all of his widely ranging researches Richet was able somehow to implicate the nervous system, including the brain. He found that fever and anaphylaxis were mediated by the brain as were the physiological and pathological effects of many toxins, anesthetics and other chemical substances. Richet's thinking about nerves and chemicals was synthesized in his remarkable 1910 address to the International Congress of Physiologists, *"L'Humorisme Ancien et l'Humorisme Moderne"*, in which he foresaw chemical neurotransmission.[R 509]

Richet's contemporary, Michael Foster, professor of physiology at Cambridge, had also recognized the fundamental importance of the nervous system as the ultimate regulator of visceral function. According to Geison, Foster insisted that the nervous system was the most important branch of physiology and quoted his comment that "the rest of physiology, judged either from a practical or theoretical point of view, is a mere appendage" (Geison 1978).

Richet's Contributions—An Assessment

Richet frequently used the term "passionné" in referring to his interest in physiology and yet, as noted earlier, there was no single line of scientific inquiry that exclusively held his interest and focused his efforts over a prolonged period. As his grandson, Gabriel, commented, "of his many, often creative, projects he thoroughly studied only a few, notably, the gastric juice, metabolic and neurophysiological experiments and anaphylaxis." Accordingly most of Richet's experiments were not subjected to tests of validity or challenged with alternate hypotheses. Nevertheless, as reflected in the methodological descriptions in his studies of fermentation, his experimental techniques were precise and meticulously applied.

Richet's longest sustained efforts in the laboratory were focused on lactic fermentation and oxidative metabolism, both central concerns of his two greatest scientific heroes, Pasteur and Lavoisier. These topics had also engaged numerous investigators in France and elsewhere in Europe, especially Germany. Although Richet's investigations yielded some original observations, his results were not such as to formulate fundamental principles or to greatly accelerate progress in either the field of fermentation (enzymology) or metabolism.

On the other hand he exploited with distinction his unique opportunity to make direct observations on gastric juice and gastric sensation in his fistulous subject, Marcellin. For that work at age twenty-nine he won the prize for experimental physiology awarded each year by the Académie des Sciences.

Richet's other original contributions, some of which had far-reaching significance, were made in areas that were not particularly popular among physiologists at the time. The special feature of these studies was Richet's remarkable insight into the biological significance of his observations. In the case of chloralose, for example, still a favored anesthetic in neurophysiological research, Richet deduced that it enhanced medullary reflexes. His inference was made before it was possible to record from neurons in situ in the brain but, as the late Albert Fessard, recording with modern techniques from the ventrolateral nucleus of the cat, acknowledged: "chloralose helps to identify these neurons and their characteristic afferent patterns by apparently lowering their firing threshold (hence enhancing medullary reflexes)" (Fessard 1976).

Richet's work on the development of bacterial resistance to metallic poisons was entirely original and, although of relatively little interest at the time, his observation gained considerable significance many years later after the discovery of antibiotics. By that time, however, Richet's unique contribution had been forgotten and was not mentioned in the address of either Monod, Jacob, or Lwoff when in 1965 they accepted the Nobel Prize for work that included the explanation of the mechanism of bacterial resistance to antibiotics (Sourkes 1966).

Another original discovery, and one of which Richet was most proud, concerned the reflex nature of panting in dogs and its importance in body temperature regulation. Related to this was his discovery that the fever of infection is mediated in the mid-brain. The direction of research in the field of heat production and heat loss at that time, however, was not toward control by the central nervous system, but toward investigations of internal combustion and circulatory behavior. By the time Barbour (Barbour 1912) and Isenschmid and Krehl (Isenschmid & Krehl 1912) in 1912 demonstrated that the trigger for the production of fever was located in the hypothalamic region of the brain, Richet's early experiment in which he induced fever by needling that area had been forgotten.

Likewise Richet's decisive experiments on oxygen conservation in diving ducks had little interest for other investigators at the time, but they became fundamental to an understanding of neural mechanisms involved in protection against hypoxia (lack of sufficient oxygen). In this case Richet's contribution was acknowledged by Laurence Irving in his important experiments forty years after Richet's studies (Irving 1934).

In these and other investigations of potential importance Richet failed to delve deeply enough. In the case of anaphylaxis, however, although he was not the first to observe the phenomenon he was certainly the first to appreciate its significance. He followed up his observation with a thorough, systematic study of anaphylaxis that extended over twelve years and yielded a distinguished contribution to medical science. Not only did Richet recognize the importance of a surprising phenomenon that had been noted casually from time to time by others in the past, but reproduced it, defined its characteristics with great care, delineated the timing and circumstances of its occurrence and of its gradual mitigation and ultimate disappearance. He also assigned it a name derived from the Greek. He further established the important point that the characteristics of anaphylaxis were not those of the chemical agent that elicited it but were distinct and uniform irrespective of the inciting agent.[R 543]

In an appraisal of the significance of his contributions to physiology, Richet might not get high marks for originality in the selection of topics for study. Neither would he be given extra credit for elegance and thoroughness in pursuing his discoveries. On the other hand he would certainly score well for repeatedly having seen in his experiments relationships that had eluded other workers, and for having synthesized and formulated biological principles that anticipated discoveries of future scientists. Moreover, although diffuseness and opportunism seemed to characterize Richet's investigative activities, there was an underlying conceptual theme that tied them together, namely his concept of disease and healing as defense of the organism governed by genetic expression and physiological adaptations to perturbations of all sorts controlled by the nervous system. Walter Cannon acknowledged that Richet's concept had anticipated the Cannon theory of homeostasis (Cannon 1926).

In his *Dictionnaire de Physiologie* Richet wrote a twenty-one-page chapter under the title "Defense (Fonctions de)."[R 419] In it he emphasized the importance of the brain and spinal cord in organizing behavioral and reflex defensive and protective responses of "internal" organs as well as "external" muscles. He cited his early experiments with the claws and tail of the crayfish, his later studies of respiration, metabolism, and body temperature control and even his Nobel prize-winning discovery of anaphylaxis as portraying defensive behavior of the body regulated by the nervous system. Among important examples were his demonstration, little noted at the time, that the body's metabolic adjustments are under regulation of the brain as is the fever of infection which is instituted by a chemical effect on the brain initiated in response to an invasion.[R 419] In his later work he showed that even the manifestations of anaphylaxis, including collapse of arterial pressure, are triggered in the brain by the combination of a tiny concentration of the offending chemical with a substance in the patient's blood serum.[R 543] Moreover, Richet was among the first to perceive the importance and the widespread effects on bodily structures of what we now call neurotransmitters, small amounts of regulatory chemicals that make the link that allows information to travel from one nerve cell to another or from nerve to gland or other tissue. In his 1910 address to the International Congress of Physiologists he linked the ancient medical wisdom of Hippocrates to what amounted to a preview of our modern knowledge of humors, neurotransmitters and other regulatory chemicals. Citing numerous examples, he showed that minuscule amounts of chemical substances can produce major changes in the cells and tissues of the body. He then predicted that the study of such substances, endowed with powerful effects in extremely low concentration, would occupy chemists and physiologists more and more as they sought to understand the workings of the human body. "There is no need," said Richet, "to place the humoral and the nervous theory in opposition to each other." Referring to the failure of histologists, notably Pflüger, to discover nerve endings penetrating into secreting cells, Richet stated, "we need not suppose that the nervous protoplasm comes into direct contact with the glandular protoplasm. It is sufficient that a minute fermentative reaction (in the nerve terminal) act chemically upon the secreting cells. Perhaps it is by an analogous mechanism that the nerves act upon the muscles and determine their reaction." Richet's remarkable prediction preceded by about eleven years Otto Loewi's (1873-1961) discovery of acetylcholine, the first identified neurotransmitter chemical (Loewi 1921) that was ultimately shown not only to mediate the effect of the vagus nerve in slowing the heart rate, but to mediate the effect of nerves on muscles as well.[5]

There can be little doubt of Richet's scientific creativity or of his foresight. There may even have been a sort of coherence among his many endeavors, but each area was too vast to have been covered or penetrated deeply in a single lifetime. Richet's catholic interests are somewhat reminiscent of those of Benjamin Franklin who, like Richet, possessed creative energy that ranged from literature, mechanics, and the sciences to philosophy and public affairs. Also, like Richet, Franklin had clear title to important discoveries concerning, for example, electricity and the Gulf Stream. But Franklin, too, was mainly a groundbreaker.

Being a groundbreaker who did not pursue to the fullest the ramifications of his original observations and innovations may, as already suggested, have been partly responsible for the relatively small size of Richet's niche in the history of medicine. However, despite the broad scattering of his interests and activities, Richet could in no way be considered a dilettante. Although he was guilty of inconsistencies, misinterpretations, and false starts, as most theoretical scientists are, he was able to make meritorious contributions in each of his areas of endeavor, scientific, literary, aeronautic, and social. Only in medical therapeutics were his contributions mediocre. Nevertheless, as his grandson, Gabriel, pointed out, many of Richet's discoveries contributed directly to clinical medicine. Serotherapy and anaphylaxis, for example, stimulated progress in molecular and clinical immunology. Today practitioners encounter daily the numerous syndromes and diseases that arise from disorders of the immuné system and rely heavily on the laboratory tests that evolved from study of the immune phenomena.

One vivid example of the medical benefits of Richet's research that became evident only many years later was his courageous pioneering work with plasma transfusion during World War I. His early studies of hemorrhagic shock had led him to the conclusion that circulating blood volume must be permanently restored to preserve life. Salt solutions offered only a brief correction and blood transfusions frequently accompanied by adverse reactions, were not practical in combat, because in those days they were administered directly from person to person. As an alternative, Charles Richet chose fresh plasma. Therefore in 1918, at age sixty-eight, running the risk of being taken prisoner, he set up the necessary equipment and infused wounded soldiers with plasma in the trenches. When the war ended his foresighted efforts were forgotten. Plasma transfusion was not revived until another war in 1943.

Others of Richet's contributions from the laboratory have had lasting clinical significance. His publications are still frequently cited in the world biomedical literature. In 1987, for example, there were citations to his book *La Chaleur Animal*, and to his articles on muscle contractures, his anthropological studies of brain weight, the post-mortem formation of urea by the liver, neural control of respiration and the dive reflex. Richet's perception that an immunologic therapy for cancer would ultimately be established has also been recently cited.

The Creative Process

In his "Patterns of Scientific Creativity" Frederick Lawrence Holmes examines the antecedents of what is often considered an unanticipated sudden flash of understanding and finds that what commonly appear to be abrupt insights are often preceded by a long intellectual struggle with an idea (Holmes 1986). As with the jigsaw puzzle, when enough parts have been assembled, the solution suddenly seems obvious. Holmes points out that the process of struggle often involves a series of trial and error arguments based on analogy.

Richet's ability to see relationships that had eluded others seems to fit a different paradigm. Although his reasoning was often based on analogy, there is little evidence of a perception being preceded by a long period of intellectual struggle. Repeatedly, to an unexpected or disappointing finding in an experiment, Richet responded as if he thought nature was trying to tell him something if he would only listen. He was quick to regroup his thoughts, change his hypothesis and shape his experiment toward a new idea. With remarkable frequency he was able to come up with a new observation or a seminal theory. Bernard before him had declared that there is no such thing as a negative experiment, only one that did not turn out as planned, but may thereby yield new information (Bernard 1952). Time after time Richet began investigations with an hypothesis that proved to be wrong, and yet for him the failure of his original idea provided a fresh clue from which he was able to identify a previously unrecognized physiological mechanism. His discovery of the heat regulating function of a dog's panting is the clearest example and, interestingly, it was the discovery that Richet considered his most original.

In his book, *The Sociology of Science*, Robert Merton described a "serendipity pattern" in science that resembles closely the process that Thomas Kuhn describes as leading to paradigms (Kuhn 1970). The sequence consists of "observing an *unanticipated, anomalous*, and *strategic* datum which becomes the occasion for developing a new theory or for extending an existing theory" (Merton 1977). The "serendipity pattern" seems to characterize many of Richet's accomplishments in physiology. Over and over in his work, like Sherlock Holmes closing in on the solution of a murder, Richet fixed on an *unanticipated* observation that was *anomalous* and that he considered important to pursue because it did not fit current assumptions and which, like one of Sherlock Holmes' clues that did not fit the otherwise plausible solution to the crime, turned out to be *strategic* because it led to fresh understanding.

Richet's discovery of passive immunization or serotherapy, as he called it, is illustrative. He and Héricourt were trying to transfer a tumor from one animal to another with the idea that cancer might be infectious. When the recipient animal developed only a staphylococcal abscess they switched their course and succeeded in protecting rabbits against fatal staphylococcal septicemia with an injection of the blood serum of the dog with the original abscess.

Although the concept was less original, the method less elegant, and the conclusion less decisive than his work on thermoregulation, Richet to the end of his life considered his discovery of what he called serotherapy to be his most important contribution to medicine. He nevertheless is not recognized today for having introduced passive immunization, the protection against specific infectious diseases through the injection of immune serum of a convalescent.

In addition to his ability to grasp an unanticipated finding and shift his focus to a more fruitful hypothesis, Richet possessed a strong intuitive quality, perhaps most clearly evident in his attempt to design an aeroplane capable of powered flight. As the celebrated mathematician and engineer Paul Painlevé, who had served as minister of aviation in the French government before becoming prime minister, concluded in the "homage" portion of the 1926 jubilee for Richet (Pettit 1926): "It was in 1890, at a time when the few advocates of air travel were regarded as ridiculous dreamers, that he [Richet] built his first airplane equipped with an internal combustion engine, but without a pilot, that attained a height of six meters.

"I remember that time and I must confess, that I gave very little attention to Richet's first publications. How could this physiologist, equipped with very little knowledge of mathematics make a serious contribution to the solution of a problem that poses the greatest mechanical challenge man has encountered? Only after a few years, during his later trials, did I realize the intuitive power of this man—the triumph of intuition is what distinguishes Richet's entire work."

Richet's creative powers in science were recognized very clearly in a tribute by Sir Charles Sherrington, who is considered by many as the father of neurophysiology. For the 1912 celebration of Richet's twenty-five years as a professor he wrote, "To honor him is to honor the spirit of physiology in its most graceful, most eloquent and most inspiring presentment—physiology poetized so to say. May we not say that there is not one whose physiological writings and speaking display such imaginative power without allowing imagination to add or to subtract from scientific truth by one iota" (Sherrington 1912).

Literary Accomplishments

Richet's interest in literature began long before he committed his career to physiology, but his most successful and significant poetry and plays were written during his years as professor. In his *Souvenirs d'un Physiologiste* he made an apology for taking time away from his work in physiology but took comfort in the fact that the great Swiss physiologist Albrecht Haller was well known for his poems, that Claude Bernard had written a dramatic tragedy, and that Charles Nicolle, a fellow Nobel Laureate in physiology and medicine, wrote novels.[R 736]

Richet's literary endeavors were serious and his poetry was of high quality. The celebrated French poet Sully-Prudhomme wrote the forward to Richet's book of fables. In it he stated that, "In reality the organ of our art is not the ear alone since poetry has rhythm it does not rely only on hearing. It is more appropriately seen as the language of the heart."[R 794] Richet's poetry was analyzed in a short paper by René Mainot, who emphasized the romantic idealism, commenting that "Richet's poetry has a deep moral flavor reflecting a strong belief in life and the destiny of man" (Mainot 1926).

Richet devoted fifty-five pages of his *Mémoires* to an uninterrupted account of his literary work. In conclusion he wrote, "I am confident that in all of my writings I have been inspired by a love of truth, of justice, and of my fellow man."

In a volume commemorating the fiftieth anniversary of Charles Richet's discovery of anaphylaxis, Professor Leon Binet, who had succeeded Henri Roger, the successor of Richet as professor of physiology, paraphrased the dictum of the writer and critic, Rémy de Gourmont,[6] "Charles Richet was one of those who enjoyed introducing literature into science and science into literature" (Binet 1952). In an obituary note his publisher George J.B. Baillière wrote, "Richet ennobled the French language discerning its nuances and selecting the proper word for clear expression" (Baillière 1935).

On the strength of his poetry and theater pieces, which had attracted acclaim from literary pundits and from the Académie Française itself for his book of fables and his poem about Pasteur, Richet presented himself twice as a candidate for membership in the Académie. Both times he was denied admission, and after that made no further attempts to qualify for membership. According to Robert Tocquet, one of his colleagues in the

Institut Métapsychique International, the reasons for refusal were that
some members of the Academy objected to Richet's pacifism, others to
vivisection and still others to his interest in psychic phenomena (Tocquet
1969). Another factor that may have been of prime importance, according
to his grandson Gabriel, was his declared agnosticism. While those who
were not religiously observant, and even anticlerics could be tolerated
by the powerful conservative element in the Académie Française, overt
agnosticism could not.

Richet's achievements should not be measured by the honors he
accumulated during his lifetime or even by the size of his niche in history
but by whether or not he accomplished what he set out to do. The
seventeenth-century *Libre pensuers* seem to have been the source of his
inspiration as transmitted through their eighteenth-century intellectual
progeny, Diderot, Condillac, and Cabanis. Jean Louis Faure's apt char-
acterization of Richet as a "free spirit" suggests that his importance and
influence should not be defined solely by criteria applicable to either a
medical scientist, a poet, novelist, playwright, historian, bibliophile,
bibliographer, aircraft designer, psychologist or philosopher. A broader
scale is required. To win a gold medal in a decathlon it is not necessary
for an athlete to place first in any single event. Richet had chosen a career
in physiology but it failed to afford him full self-expression. He wanted
to excel in many endeavors in preference to investing himself exclusively
in one. His close friend, Emile Gley (1926) characterized Richet's
aspirations by paraphrasing a couplet about Icarus from Ovid's *Meta-
morphoses*:

He lived pursuing a high adventure
The sky was his desire . . .

In this respect Richet may seem to share some of the characteristics of a
"golden boy." Golden boys are multitalented achievers whose aim is to
excel without being greatly concerned about the nature of the challenge.
Their implicit message is "To win I need only to know the goal and the
rules." Like Richet, most golden boys are articulate, charming, and
resourceful but they usually possess an emotional invulnerability that
Richet did not share. Thus golden boys usually lack a clear and consum-
ing commitment for which they are willing to sacrifice other gains. Here,
again, the pattern of the golden boy clearly does not fit Richet. Richet
was deeply committed to his goals and prepared to make sacrifices for
them. He aspired not only to contribute to physiology and literature, but

to France, to peace, to the alleviation of human suffering and the improvement of the human race. His desire to achieve in these and other areas as well seemed to create in him a troubling ambivalence and inner struggle as suggested by his poem, *Jeannot Lapin* and the reverie that he called *Two Voices in a Dream*. Although the final verses of *Jeannot Lapin* are directed to his children with the explanation that his message was a plea for peace and a rejection of political tyrants, the fact that he used as a model a savant conducting an experiment with vivisection suggests an unconscious conflict about his career. *Two Voices in a Dream* reveals even more clearly his doubts about having continually interrupted his laboratory work for causes and literary activities.

Despite such despondent reflections Richet could take heart from the judgment of his contemporaries expressed in the homage portion of his 1926 festschrift. The keynote speaker, Felix Luis Henneguy (1850–1928) president of the Société de Biologie declared, "You have not been content to be a great biologist. In a period of decadence that we are going through because the humanities are considered useless and undemocratic, you have been able to bring arts and letters together with science; as a poet, historian, moralist and philosopher, you are accorded a place of high honor among the most cultivated of men."

In 1987, celebrating the 100th anniversary of Richet's accession to the Chair of Physiology at the Faculté de Médecine in Paris, the French government issued a commemorative postage stamp.

Notes

1. Richet was deeply sympathetic with the seemingly endless suffering of the Poles, their country having been violated and partitioned over and over again for centuries. On a visit to Russia during World War I he encountered many Polish refugee families who had escaped the Germans. "They had a vague feeling that the moment of their liberation was approaching," he wrote, "I visited them frequently and received a welcome of more warmth and tenderness than I have ever experienced except, perhaps, in France" (Unp).
2. Cuvier opposed the views of the earlier philosophers and natural scientists, Johann Wolfgang von Goethe, Friedrich Wilhelm Joseph von Schelling (1775–1854) and Keilmayer, especially the latter's view that any whole creature, plant or animal, is identified by the balance of polarities, intake and outflow, positive and negative, etc. To Cuvier the concept of organism implied that all its parts were independent, interactive and contributory to the whole. He also rejected the ideas of Benoit de Maillet (1656–1738) and Lamarck that parts or features of living beings were shaped by their endeavor. Cuvier recognized an inherent capacity of all parts to evolve, grow, and function in a unified fashion (Cuvier 1831).

3. The letters were edited and published as a book.[R 428] Richet contended that the concept of purpose translates into the will to survive. Sully-Prudhomme further developed the idea in the framework of evolution in an attempt to reconcile metaphysics with sciences that deal with the tangible.

4. Loeb (1859–1924) an almost militant mechanist, was deeply interested in the inheritance of separate characteristics through genetic mutation. In his book, *The Organism as a Whole*, he praised Darwin for "his insistence that accidental, and not purposeful variations gave rise to the organisms." Loeb believed that the harmonious working together of the organs and tissues of a living being is also genetically determined but he was skeptical of Darwin's proposal of "adaptation" with its unacceptable implications of purpose (Loeb 1916).

5. Michael Foster, also in anticipation of Otto Loewi's experimental demonstration of neurotransmission, had suggested that the vagus nerve exerts its inhibition on the heart rate by chemical mediation. Foster's colleagues, John Newport Langley (1857–1925) and Walter Holbrook Gaskell (1847–1917) extended the idea of chemical mediation of nerve impulses in the sympathetic nerves supplying the heart which they called the "katabolic accelerators" (Langley 1921, Gaskell 1916).

6. "Il faut faire entrer le plus possible de littérature dans la science, et de science dans la littérature." (Gourmont 1926).

References

Ackerknecht, E. H. 1967. *Medicine at the Paris Hospital 1749-1848.* Baltimore: Johns Hopkins Press.

Altschule, M. 1984. *Science and Medicine in France. The Emergence of Experimental Physiology, 1790-1855, John E. Lesch,* p. 276. Cambridge: Harvard University Press.

Andersen, H. T. 1963. "The reflex nature of the physiological adjustments to diving and their afferent pathways." *Archives Internal Medicine,* 58:263.

Anderson, J. F. and M. J. Rosenau. 1909. "Anaphylaxis." *Archives Internal Medicine* 3:519-568 (Lecture Delivered before the Harvey Society, December 5, 1908).

Arohnson, E., Sachs, S. 1886. "Die Beziehungen des Gehirns zur Körperwärme und zum Fieber: Experimentelle Untersuchungen. *Archives für Gesampte Physiologie.* (Pflügers) 37:232-299.

Arthus, M. 1921. *L'Anaphylaxie à L'Immunité.* Paris: Masson.

Auer, J. 1910. "The prophylactic action of atropin in immediate anaphylaxis of guinea pigs." *American Journal of Physiology,* 27, 439-452.

Aufderheide, K. 1980. "Cellular Aspects of Pattern Formation—The Problem of Assembly." *American Journal of Physiology,* 44:252-303.

Baillière, J. B. G. 1935. "Charles Richet (1850-1935)" *Necrologie des Practiciers,* Paris.

Baldwin, R. W., Byers, V. S. 1986. "Monoclonal antibodies in cancer treatment." *Lancet* March 15, 2:603.

Barbour, H. G. 1912. "Die Wirkung Unmittelbarer Erwärmung und Abkulhung der Wärmezentra auf die Körpertemperatur." Nauyn-Schmiedberg: *Archives Experimental Pathologie Pharmakologie.* 70:1-26.

Beaumont, W. 1833. *Experiments and observations on the gastric juice and physiology of digestion.* Plattsburg: F.P. Allen.

Bernard, C. 1839. *Des Liquids de l'Organisme* tome III, p. 46, Paris: Baillière.

Bernard, C. 1856. *Leçon de Physiologie Expérimentale Appliqué à la Médicine* Paris: Baillière (2 vols).

Bernard, C. 1952. *An Introduction to the Study of Experimental Medicine.* New York: Henry Schumann.

Bernheim, H. 1889. *Suggestive Therapeutics. A treatise on the nature and uses of hypnotism.* English translation by C.A. Herter, New York: G.P. Putnam & Sons.

Bert, P. 1879. *Leçons sur la physiologie comparée de la respiration.* Paris: Baillière.

Besredka, A., Bronfenbrenner, J. 1911. "De l'anaphylaxie et de l'antianaphylaxie. vis-a-vis du Blanc D'oeuf." *Annals de l'Institute Pasteur.* XXV:392-414.

Besredka, A. 1917. *Anaphylaxie et anti anaphylaxie; bases expérimentales,* préfaces de E. Roux, Paris: Masson & Cie.

Binet, L. 1952. "L'anaphylaxie (Travail redigé pour le cinquantenaire de la decouverte de Ch. Richet et P. Portier." *Presse Médicale*, 60:683-695.

Borelli, G. A. 1681. *De Motu Animalism.* vol. 1 & II, Rome: Bernabo.

Bouquet, H. 1935. "Chronique sur Charles Richet." *Le Monde Médicale*, Jan. 1, 24-27.

Breguet, C. A. J. 1980. "The Breguet Dynasty—Two centuries of interdisciplinary scientists—engineers." *Interdisciplinary Science Review*, 5 (2):149-164.

Brobeck, J. R. (Ed). 1973. *Best & Taylor's Physiological Basis of Medical Practice*, (9th edition) Baltimore: Williams & Wilkins.

Cabanis, J. P. G. 1981. In *On the Relations Between the Physical and Moral Aspects of Man*: 1:31-79, edited by G. Mora, vol. 1, Baltimore: Johns Hopkins University Press.

Cannon, W. B. 1926. In *Charles Richet, Ses Amis, ses Colléques, ses Elèves* Pettit A. ed., Paris, Imperimerie des Editions Médicales, pp. 91-93.

Carnot, N. L. 1824. *Reflexions sur la Puissance Motrice du Feu et sur les Machines Propres à Developer cette Puissance.* London: R.A. Thurston.

Carvallo, J. L. 1902. "Estomac", In: Richet, C. *Dictionnaire de Physiologie*, vol. 5, pp. 849-854.

Carvallo, J. L. 1911. *Thèse. Le Doctorate en Médecine. Methode Radiochronophotographique.* Paris: Masson.

Cesalpino, A. 1571. *Quaestinam Peripateticarum.* Libri Quinque. Venetius, Iuntas.

Chamberland, C. E. 1887. "Annales de l'Institut Pasteur;" cited in *Dictionnaire de Physiologie*, vol. 1, p. 606.

Charcot, J. L. M. 1878. "Catalepsie et somnambulisme, hysteriques, provoqués." Cited by A.R.G. Owen, In *Hysteria, Hypnosis and Healing*, 1971, London, Dennis Dobson, p.185.

Condillac, E. B. 1752. In *Diderot, D. 1751-1780*.

Encyclopédie, out Dictionnaire Raissonné des Sciences, des arts et des Métiers (35 vols) Neuchatel, vol., 8, 741-3.

Cornax, M. 1564. "Medical consultationis apud aegrotos secundum artem et experientiam salubriter instituendae enchiridion." Bale. Cited by C.J. Cumston, *Medical Journal & Record* 124:299, 1926.

Corvisart, J. N., Leroux, J. J. 1802. "Observations sur une ouverture fistuleuse à l'estomac." *Journal Medicine Chirurgie et Pharmacologie.* 111: 407.

Cuvier, G. 1831. *The Animal Kingdom.* vol. 1, G, C & H, New York: Carvill.

d'Arsonval, J. A. 1894. "L'anemo-calorimetrie ou nouvelle méthode de calorimetrie humaine normal et pathologique." *Archives de Physiologie* (5) vol. 1, 360-390, & B.B. (9) vol. 1, 77.

Darwin, C. 1859. *Origin of Species.* New York: P.F. Collier & Son.

Davis, B. B. 1967. "Metabolic Regulation and Information Storage in Bacteria." In Quarton, G.C., Melenecheck, T. and F.O. Schmitt (Eds): *The Neurosciences.* New York: Rockefeller University Press, 114-115.

Degler, C. N. 1990. *In Search of Humane Nature. The Decline and Revival of Darwinism in American Social Thought.* Oxford University Press, NY.

De Land, F. H. 1989. "A perspective of monoclonal antibodies: past, present and future." *Seminars in Nuclear Medicine,* 3:158-165.

Dewhurst, K. 1963. *John Locke (1632-1704). Physician and Philosopher. A Medical Biography.* London: Wellcome History Medical Library.

Dubos, R. 1950. In *Louis Pasteur. Free Lance of Science.* Boston: Little Brown & Co.

Duffin, J. 1988. "Vitalism and Organicism in the Philosophy of R.T.H. Laennec." *Bulletin History of Medicine,* 62:4, 527.

Ehrlich, P. 1897. "Zur Kenntriss der Antitoxinwirkung." *Fortsch. der Medizin.* 15 January.

Ehrlich, P. 1907. "Chemotherapeutische Trypanosomen Studien." *Berliner Klinische Wochenschrift,* 9-12.

Elsner, R., Gooden, B. A. 1970. "Reduction of reactive hyperemia on the human forearm by face immersion." *Journal Applied Physiology,* 29:627-630.

Faure, J. L. 1935. "Paroles prononcées aux obseques de Charles Richet." *Presse médicale,* 43:2023-2024, December 11.

Feinstein, R., Pinsker, H., Schmale, M., and B. A. Gooden. 1977. "Bradycardial response in aplysia exposed to air." *Journal Comparative Physiology* 122:311-324.

Fessard, A. 1976. "Sur la complexité d'hierarchisée du systeme nerveux et ses modeles d'organization." *Review Electroenceph. Neurophysiol. Clin.* 6(4)481-487.

Fielding, E., Baggally, W. W., and Carrington, H. 1909. *Society for Psychical Research Proceedings,* 25:309.

Flexner, R. 1912. "Medical Education in Europe." A Report to the Carnegie Foundation for the Advancement of Teaching. New York.

Foster, M. 1899. "Claude Bernard." In *The Masters of Medicine,* New York: Longmans.

Fox, R., Weisz, G. 1980. *The Organization of Science and Technology in France 1804-1914,* Cambridge: Cambridge University Press.

Fye, B. 1986. "Sir Lauder Brunton and Amyl Nitrite: A Victorian Vasodilator." *Circulation,* 74:222-229.

Galvani, L. 1981. "Sixth memoir. On the Influence of the temperaments on the formation of the moral ideas and affections." In *On the Relations of the Physiological and Moral Aspects of Man.* by Cabanis, J.G., vol. 1, pp. 265-313. Baltimore: Johns Hopkins University Press.

Gaskell, W. H. 1916. *The Involuntary Nervous System.* London: Longmans, Green & Co.

Geison, G. L. 1978. *The Cambridge School of Psychology.* Princeton: Princeton University Press.

Gley, E. 1926. "Charles Richet Physiologiste." *Progrès Médicale,* 21:792-803.

Gourmont, R de. 1926. "Quoted by E. Callamand de Sainte-Mande." *Progrès Médicale,* No. 6, Supplement Illustré.

Grmek, M. D. 1966. *Bernard,C. Bibliography. Original Works. Dictionary of Scientific Biography*. Charles Coulston Gillespie, editor, vol. 4, Hans Berger, Christoph Buys Ballot, 33-34, New York: Charles Scribner's Sons.

Gunn, C. G. 1972. In *The Artery and the Process of Arteriosclerosis. Measurement & Modification*. Stewart Wolf, editor, pp. 222, New York: Plenum Press.

Hall, M. 1832. *On the reflex function of the mediulla oblongata and the medulla spinalis*. London: Bailliere.

Hartman, F. 1891. Translation In *Paracelsus*. John W. Lowell Co., Reprinted 1963 by Health Research, Mohlumne Hill, CA.

Harvey, W. 1628. *Exercitatio Anatomea de Motu Cordus at Sanguinis in Animalibus*. Francfort, Fitzeri.

Heidenhain, R. 1880. *Animal Magnetism, Physiological Observations*. London: Woolridge.

Helm, J. 1801. "Geschichte einer ubrigens gesunden person mit einem von aussen sichtbaren Loche in Magen." *Gesundheitstaschen Buch. fur das Jahr*, Wien: 241-245.

Helmholz, H. Von. 1847. *Uber die Erhaltung der Krafte*. Berlin: Reimer.

Hermann, H. 1859. "De tono et moto musculorum nonnulla." *Archives fur des Gesampte Physiologie*. (Pflügers), 13:369.

Hoffman, A. 1898. "Stoffwechseluntersuchungen nach totaler Magenresection."

Holmes, F. L. 1974. *Claude Bernard and Animal Chemistry*. Commonwealth Fund: Harvard University Press.

Holmes, F. L. 1975. "Review of Charles R. Richet." In *Dictionnary of Scientific Biography*, vol. XI, 425-431, New York: Charles Scribner.

Holmes, F. L. 1986. "Patterns of Scientific Creativity. The Fielding Garrison Lecture." *Bulletin History of Medicine*, 60:19-35.

Irving, L. 1934. "On the ability of warm blooded animals to survive without breathing." *Science Monthly*, 38:422-428.

Isenschmid, R., Krehl, L. 1912. "Ueber den Einfluss des Gehirns aus die warmeregulation." *Archives fur Experimental Pathologie & Pharmakologie* 70:109-134.

James, L. S. 1958. Rept. Ross Pediatric Research Conf. of 1958, p. 66.

Janet, P. 1923. "A propos de la métapsychique." *Revue Philosophique*, 96:5-32.

Johnson, S. P. 1968. *Encyclopedia Brittanica* 2:901-913.

Jones, S. 1875. "Gastrostomy for structure (cancerous?) of esophagus, death from bronchitis 40 days after operation." *Lancet* 1:678.

Juri, M. 1965. "On Richet, Charles Richet Physiologiste, 1850-1935." *Zürcher Medizingeschichtliche Abhandlungen* 34:7-47.

Kennedy, E. 1979. "Ideology" from Destutt de Tracy to Marx." *Journal History of Ideology*, 40:353-368.

Kuhn, T. S. 1970. *"The Structure of Scientific Revolutions."* Chicago: University of Chicago Press.

Lagarde, A., Michard, L. 1955. *XIXe Sicle*, Paris: Bordas, pp. 393.

Langley, J. N. 1921. *The Autonomic Nervous System*. Part 1, Cambridge: Heffer & Sons.

Langlois, J. P. 1906. "Les Recherches récentes sur la fièvre des foins." *Presse Médicale* 14:583.

Lesch. J. E. 1977. *The Origins of Experimental Physiology and Pharmacology in France: 1790–1820*. University Microfilms Institute. Ann Arbor, Michigan.

Locke, J. 1981. "An Essay Concerning Human Understanding." A.C. Campbell, ed., Oxford Claredon Press, 2 vols.

Loeb, J. 1916. "The Organism as a Whole and from a Physicochemical Viewpoint." New York: G.P. Putnam Sons.

Loewi, O. 1921. "Uber humorale ubertragbargen der hertznervenwirkung." *Archives fur des Gesampte Physiologie* 189:239-242.

Loir, A. 1926. "Une suite au jubilé de Prof. Chas. Richet." *La Vie Médicale*, 2397-2398, November 11.

Longcope, N. T. 1943. "Foreword to Maurice Arthus' Philosophy of Scientific Investigation." Trans. from French with an introduction by H. Sigerist. *Bulletin History of Medicine* 14:366-390.

Longet, F. A. 1860-1861. *Traité de Physiologie*, Paris: F. Alcan.

Luchsinger, C. 1882. *Archives fur des Gesampte Physiologie* 28:60.

Magendie, F. 1839. *Leçons sur les Fonctions et les Maladies du Systéme Nerveux*. Paris: Ebrard.

Mainot, R. 1926. "Propose du Jour. Critique du Poesie de Charles Richet." *La Vie Médicale* 2127-2128, September 15.

Malpighi, M. 1661. "Duae Epistolae de Pulmonibas." Florence. (Quoted in M. Foster. 1901, Lectures on the History of Physiology. London: Cambridge University Press).

Malpighi, M. 1661. "Duae Epistolae de Pulmonibas." Florence. (Quoted in L.G. Wilson, 1959, Erasistratus, Galen and the pneuma. *Bulletin History of Medicine*, 33(4): 293-314

Mauskopf, S. H., McVaugh, M. R. 1980. *The Elusive Science. Origins of Experimental Psychical Research*. Baltimore: Johns Hopkins University Press.

Mayer, A. 1936. "Notice necrologique sur M. Charles Richet Séance Du." *Bulletin Académie de Médecine.*, New York: Henry Schumann, pp. 51-64, January 14.

Mayer, J. P. 1948. *The Recollections of Alexis de Tocqueville*. Trans. by Alexander Teixeira de Mattos. London: The Harvell Press.

Mayer, J. R. Von. 1842. "Bemerkungen über die Krafte der unbelebter Natur." *Annals Chemical U. Pharmacologie* 42:233-240.

Merton, R. K. 1977. *The Sociology of Science*. Carbondale & Edwardsville: Southern Illinois University Press.

Metchnekoff, E. 1901. *L'immunite dans les Maladies Infectueuses*. Paris: Masson.

Moulin, A. M. 1989. "The Immune system: A Key Concept for the History of Immunology." *History Philosophical Life Sciences*. 11:221–236.

Müller, J. 1834–40. *Handbuch der Physiologie des Menschen for Vorlesungen*. Cablenz, J. Holscher.

Nock, J. 1934. *A Journey into Rabelais' France*. New York: William Morris & Co., p. 303.

Olmsted, J. M. D. 1938. *Claude Bernard, physiologist*. New York: Harper & Brothers.

Olmsted, J. M. D., Olmsted, E. H. 1952. *Claude Bernard and the Experimental Method in Medicine*. New York: Henry Schumann.

Osler, W. 1943. "The Master Word in Medicine." In *Aequinimitas with other addresses*. chap. 10, pp. 347, 3rd edition. Philadelphia: The Blakiston Co.

Osty, E. 1936. "Charles Richet (1850–1935)." *Revue Métaphysique* Jan-Feb. de l'Instut Métaphysique International.

Owen, A. R. G. 1971. *Hysteria, hypnosis and healing: The world of J.M. Charcot*, London: Dobson Books.

Pachon, V. 1907. "Sur la Résistance Comparée du Canard et du Pigeon a l'asphyxie dans l'air Confiné." *Société de Biologie Séance Du*. Paris, June 15, pp 1120–1123.

Pachon, V. 1912. "Une orientation nouvelle la sphygmomanométrie. La presson minima considerée comme base de sphygommanometrie." *Melanges Biologiques*. Paris: Imprimerie de la Cour d'Appel.

Paracelsus. 1891. "De Moto Pharmacandi," In *Paracelsus*. Translated by F. Hartman. John W. Lowell. Reprinted 1963 by Health Research, Mohlumne Hill, CA.

Paul, H. 1985. *From Knowledge to Power*. Cambridge University Press: NY.

Perkins, J. F. 1964. "Historical development of Respiratory Physiology" IN Fenn, W.O. & Rahn, H. *Handbook of Physiology*, Washington, Amer. Physiol. Soc., pp. 1–62.

Pettit, A. 1926. *Sérothapie anti-poliomyélitique*. Jubilé Charles Richet. Paris: Editions Médicales.

Pettenkofer, M. 1862. "Ueber die Respiration." *Annals Chimique U. Pharmacologie Supplement* 2:1–52.

Pieron, H. 1922. "Revue (Traité de Métapsychique)." *L'Année Psychologique* 23:602.

Pierson, J. 1940. "Charles Richet. His attitude and influence on psychical research in Europe." *Journal American Society for Psychical Research*, vol. XXV: 6:173–183, June.

Prout, W. 1824. "On the nature of the acid and saline matters usually existing in the stomach of animals." *Philosophical Transactions* 114:45.

Raine, C. S. (Ed.). 1988. *Advances in Neuroimmunology*. New York Academy of Sciences, Annals, vol. 540.

Regnault, H. V., Reiset, F. 1849. "Recherches chimiques sur la respiration des animaux de diverses classes." *Annales Chimique et Physiologique* 26:299.

Renan, E. 1863. "Vie de Jesus." *Histoire des Origines de Christianisme*. Paris: 18th Century Book.

Richard, L., Richet-Papier. 1910. "Archives du Musée Oceanographique de Monaco."

Richer, P., Charcot, J. M. 1883. *Contributions à l'étude de l'hypnotisme chez les hysteriques*. Paris: A. Delahaye et Lecrosnier.

Richet, A. 1855-1857. *Traite Pratique d'Anatomie Chirurgicale*. VIII:1026, Paris: F. Chamerot.

Richet, A. 1864. "Recherches sur les tumeurs vasculaires des os, dites tumeurs fongueuses sanguines des os ou aneurysmes des os." *Archives Génerale de Médicine* Paris: P. Asselin, 80.

Richet, Charles Fils. 1957. *Pathologie de la Misère*. Paris: Société de Diffusion Médicale et Scientifique.

Robertson, J. M. Cited in Fellows, O.E. and N.L. Torrey. 1971. *The Age of Enlightenment*. 2nd ed. New York: Appleton Century Crofts, p. 7.

Robin, E. D., Murdaugh, H. V. 1963. "Adaptation to diving in the Harbor Seal-gas exchange and ventilatory response to CO_2." *American Journal Physiology* 205(6):1175-1177.

Rosenau, M. J., Anderson, J. F. 1906. "Hypersusceptibility." (Abstract) *JAMA*, vol. 13.

Roux, E., Yersin, A. 1888. "Contributions to the Studies of Diphtheria." *Annals de l'Institute Pasteur*, pp. 629-661.

Rubner, M. 1894. "Die Quelle der Thierischen Wärme." *Zeitschrift fur Biologie*, 30:73.

Schneider, W. H. 1986a. "Puericulture and the style of French Eugenics." *Historical Philosophical Life Sciences* 8:265-277.

Schneider, W. H. 1986b. *Charles Richet and the Social Role of Medical Men*. Presented at the 32nd Annual Meeting of the Society for French Historical Studies, Quebec, March, 22.

Scholander, P. F. 1962. *Physiological Adaptations to Diving in Animals and Man*. The Harvey Lectures. New York: Academic Press Series.

Sechenov, I. 1952. *Reflexes of the Brain*. Reprinted by (I & Z-VO) Academy of Medicine, USSR: Nauk.

Sherrington, C. S. 1912. *Note on present problems of nervous function*. Jubilé du Prof. Charles Richet, Paris: L. Maretheux, pp. 40.

Sigerist, H. E. 1943. "Maurice Arthus' Philosophy of Scientific Investigations." *Bulletin History of Medicine*, 14:366-390.

Sourkes, T. L. 1966. *Nobel Prize Winners in Medicine and Physiology 1901-1965*. Abelard-Schuman.

Spallanzani, A. L. 1777. *Observations et expériences sur quelques animaux enfermé dans l'air. Opuscules de physique, animale et végétable*. 2 vols., Geneva, 236-298.

Spallanzani, A. L. 1782. "Delle digestione degli animale." Venice: *Fisica Animale*.

Strauss, H. 1903. "Zur Behandlung und Verhütung der Nierenwassersucht." *Die Therapie der Gegenwart*, Mai, 193–200.

Stromme, S. B., Kerem, D., and Elsner, R. 1970. "Diving bradycardia during rest and exercise and its relation to physical fitness." *Journal Applied Physiology*, 28:614.

Temkin, O. 1946. "Materialism in French and German Physiology of the early 19th Century." *Bulletin History of Medicine* v. 20:B-322–327.

Tocquet, R. 1969. *Charles Richet, Président de l'Institut Metapsychique Internationel*. Nouvelle, 14:9–17, June.

Vaughan, V. 1926. *A Doctor's Memories*. Indianapolis: Bobbs.

Verneuil, H. 1876. "Observation de gastro-stomie pratiquée avec succès pour un rétrécissement cicatricel infranchissable de l'oesophage." *Bulletin de l'Académie de Médecine*, Paris: 5:1023.

Von Behring, E., Kitasato, S. 1890. "Untersuchen uber des Zustandkommen Diptherie-Immunitat bei Thiere." *Deutsche med. Woch.* 6:1145–1148.

Von Mayer, J. M. 1842. "Bemerkungen where die Krafte der Unhelehten Natur." *Annals Chemistry and Pharmacology*, 42:233–240.

Whyte, L. L. 1962. *The Unconscious Before Freud*. London: Travistock Press.

Widal, F. 1905. "Les régimes déchlorés." *Rapport au Congrès Français de Médecine*, Paris: Masson.

Wolf, S., Wolff, H. 1943. *Human Gastric Function: An Experimental Study of a Man and his Stomach*. New York: Oxford University Press.

Wolf, S. 1965. "The Bradycardia of the Dive Reflex. A Possible Mechanism of Sudden Death." *Transactions American Clinical and Climatological Association*, 76:192–200.

Wolf, S. 1966. "Further studies on the circulatory and metabolic alterations of the oxygen-conserving (diving) reflex in man." *Transactions Association of American Physicians*, 78:242.

Wolf, S. 1968. "Neural mechanisms of sudden cardiac death." The Jeremiah Metzger Lecture. *Transactions American Clinical & Climatological Association*, 79:158–176.

Wolff, H. G. 1953. *Stress and Disease*. Springfield, Charles C. Thomas.

Wolff, H. G., Hardy, J. D., and Goodell, H. 1940. "Studies on pain: Measurement of the effect of morphine, codeine, and other opiates on the pain threshold and an analysis of their relation to the pain experience." *Journal Clinical Investigation*, 19:659.

Wolff, H. G., Hardy, J. D., and Goodell, H. 1941. "Measurement of the effect on the pain threshold of acetylsalicylic acid, acetanilid, acetophenetidin, aminopyrine, ethyl alcohol, trichlorethylene, a barbiturate, quinine, ergotamine tartrate and caffeine: an analysis of their relationship to the pain experience." *Journal Clinical Investigation*, 20:63.

Wright, G. L. (Ed). 1984. *Monoclonal Antibodies in Cancer*. New York: Marcel Dekker.

Wroblewski, 1898. "Eine chimische Notiz auf Schlatter's totalen Magenextirpation." *Centralblatt Ü Physiology*, 11:665–668.

Wundt, W. 1893. *Hypnotisme et Suggestion.* Translated into French by A. Keller
- Paris: Ancien Librairie Germer Baillière et Cie, F. Alcan.

Charles Richet Bibliography

1. Richet, C. 1874. La suggestion mentale et le calcul des probabilités. *Revue Scientifique*, 18:609-71.
2. Richet, C. 1875. Le somnambulisme provoqué. *Journal d'anatomie et de physiologie norm. et pathologie et l'homme et des animaux*, 11:348-78.
3. Richet, C. 1876. De l'état fonctionnel des nerfs dan l'hemianésthésie hystérique. *Comptes rendus de la Société de Biologie*, 20 Jan., 22.
4. Richet, C. 1876. De deux formes différentes de tétanos reconnues par le pneumographe. *Compte rendus de la Société de Biologie*, 4 Mar., 17-20.
5. Richet, C. 1876. Etudes sur la vitesse et les modifications de la sensibilité chez les ataxiques. *Memoires de la Société de Biologie*, 17 June, 79-89.
6. Richet, C. 1877. *Recherches Expérimentales et Cliniques sur la Sensibilité*. Paris: Masson, 342.
7. Richet, C. 1877. De l'addition latente des excitations éléctriques dans les nerfs et dans les muscles. *Travaux de Laboratoire*, de M. Marey 1. III, 97-105.
8. Richet, C. 1877. *Les Poisons de l'Intelligence*. Paris: Ollendorf.
9. Richet, C. 1877. Etude sur la douleur. *Revue Philosophique*, 21:457.
10. Richet, C. 1877. Essai sur les causes de dégout. *Revue des Deux Mondes*, 22:644-73.
11. Richet, C. 1877. De la recherche des acides libres du suc gastrique. *Comptes rendus de l'Académie des Sciences*, Paris: June, 84:1514.
12. Richet, C. 1877. De la nature des acides contenus dans le suc gastrique. *Comptes rendus de l'Académie des Sciences*, Paris: 16 July, 85:155.
13. Richet, C. 1877. Recherches sur l'acidité du suc gastrique de l'homme et observation sur la digestion stomacal faites sur une fistule gastrique. *Comptes rendus de l'Académie des Sciences*, Paris: 85:450-452.
14. Richet, C. 1878. *Du suc gastrique chez l'homme et les animaux, ses propriétés chimiques et physiologiques*, Paris: G. Baillière, 167.
15. Richet, C. 1878. Des propriétés chimiques et physiologiques du suc gastrique chez l'homme et les animaux. *Supplement Journal d'Anatomie et de la Physiologie*, 14:170.
16. Richet, C. 1878. *Structure des circonvolutions cérébrales (anatomie et physiologie). Thèse d'agrégation de la Faculté de Médecine à Paris*, G. Baillière, 175.
17. Richet, C. 1878. Sur l'acide du suc gastrique. *Comptes rendus de l'Académie des Sciences*, Paris, 4 Mar., 676.
18. Richet, C. 1878. De la fermentation lactique du sucre de choc péritonéal. *Comptes rendus de l'Académie des Sciences*, Paris: 90:1220-1223.
19. Richet, C. 1878. De l'excitabilité du muscle pendant les différentes périodes de sa contraction. Travaux du laboratoire du Prof. Vulpian, à la Faculté de Médecine, 242-24
20. Moutard-Martin, R. and C. Richet. 1879. Contribution à l'étude des injections intraveineuses de lait et de sucre. *Gazette Médecine de Paris* (6th ser.), 1:588, 600-24.

21. Richet, C. 1879. Remarques et observations physiologiques sur l'acidité du suc gastrique humain dépourv de salive. *Comptes rendus de la Société de Biologie*, Paris: (6th ser.) 4:119–24.

22. Richet, C. 1879. Contribution à la physiologie des centres nerveux et des muscles de l'écrevisse. *Archives de Physiologie norm. et Pathologie*, Paris: (2nd ser.) 6:262–99; 522–576.

23. Richet, C. 1879. De la nutrition. *Progrès Médecine*, Paris: 7:397, 477, 498, 580, 600, 659.

24. Richet, C. 1879. La métaphysique de Claude Bernard d'après Letourneau. Correspondence. *Revue Scientifique*, Paris (2nd ser.) 17:303–77.

25. Richet, C. 1879. La peste en Russie. *Revue des Deux Mondes*, Paris: 32:460–68.

26. Richet, C. 1879. La découverte de la circulation du sang.

27. Richet, C. 1879. Le congrès médical d'Amsterdam en 1879 Chir. et Pharmacol., Bux: 69:416.

28. Breguet, A. and C. Richet. 1879. De l'influence de la durée de l'intensité sur la perception lumineuse. *Comptes rendus de l'Academie des Sciences*, Paris: 88:239.

29. Richet, C. 1879. De l'excitabilité des muscles pendant les différentes périodes de la contraction. *Comptes rendus de l'Academie des Sciences*, Paris: 88:242–244.

30. Richet, C. 1879. De quelques conditions de la fermentation lactique. *Comptes rendus de l'Académie des Sciences*, Paris: 88:750–52.

31. Richet, C. 1879. De la forme de la contraction musculaire des muscles de l'écrevisse. *Comptes rendus de l'Académie des Sciences*, Paris: 28 April, 88:868.

32. Richet, C. 1879. De l'influence de la chaleur sur les fonctions des centres nerveux de l'écrevisse. *Comptes rendus de l'Académie des Sciences*, Paris: 12 May, 88:977.

33. Moutard-Martin, R., Richet, C. 1879. Influence du sucre injecté dans les veines sur la sécrétion renale. *Comptes rendus de l'Académie des Sciences*, Paris: 89:240–42; also *Journal de Médecine*.

34. Richet, C. 1879. De l'action des courants électriques sur les muscles de la pince de l'écrevisse. *Compte rendus de l'Académie des Sciences*, Paris: 89:242–44.

35. Brissaud, E., Richet, C. 1879. De quelques faits relaifs aux contractures. *Comptes rendus de l'Académie des Sciences*, Paris: 89:489–91.

36. Richet, C. 1879. De l'excitabilité rythmique des muscles et de leur comparaison avec le coeur. *Comptes rendus de l'Académie des Sciences*, Paris: 89:792–94; *Gazette Médecine de Paris* (6th ser.) 1:614.

37. Moutard-Martin, R. and C. Richet. 1879. Des causes de la mort par les injections intraveineuses de lait et de sucre. *Comptes rendus de l'Académie des Sciences*, Paris: 14 July.

38. Richet, C. 1879. *Histology and Physiology of the Cerebral Convolutions, Translated by E. Fowler and Poisons of the Intellect, Translated by John C. Minor*. New York: Wm. Wood & Co.

39. Richet, C. 1879. Chimie physiologique de la nutrition. *Progrès Médecine*, Paris.

40. Richet, C. 1879. Charles Renouard 1794–1878 Discours prononcés à la Cour de Cassation. Notice sur sa vie. Paris: P. Ollendorf.

41. Richet, C. 1879. Foreword to Harvey, W. La circulation du sang; des mouvements du coeur chez l'homme et chez les animaux; deux réponses à Riolan. Traduction Française, avec une introduction historique et des notes. Paris: G. Masson, 287.

42. Richet, C. 1880. Vivisection and its use in therapeutics and hygiene. *Lancet*, London: 1:441-43.

43. Richet, C. 1880. Recherches sur la contraction musculaire de l'écrevisse. *Cong. périod Internat. d. sc. méd. Compt. rend. Amst.* 6:554-560.

44. Richet, C. 1880. Contribution à la physiologie des centres nerveux et des muscles de l'écrevisse. *Archives de Physiologie*, 7:262-94, 522-76.

45. Breguet, A. and C. Richet. 1880. De l'influence de la durée et de l'intensité de la lumière sur la perception lumineuse. Paris: G. Masson, 689-96.

46. Brissaud, E. and C. Richet. 1880. Faits pour servir à l'histoire des contractures. *Progrès Médecine* Paris: 8:365-67, 499, 466.

47. Richet, C. 1880. De la nutrition. *Progès Médecine*, Paris: 8:1031-33.

48. Richet, C. 1880. Du somnabulisme provoqué. *Review Philosophique de la France et de l'étranger*, 10:337-484.

49. Richet, C. 1880. Hysteria and demonism; a study in morbid psychology. *Popular Science Monthly*, New York: 17:86-93; 155-65; 376-85; translated from *Revue des Deux Mondes*, Paris.

50. Berger, M.P. and C. Richet. 1880. Des travaux récents relatifs aus anesthésiques. *Revue Scientifique*, Paris: (2nd ser.) 18:1232-34.

51. Richet, C. 1880. Des mouvements de la cellule. *Revue Scientifique*, Paris: (2nd ser.) 19:458-65.

52. Richet, C. 1880. Les ètudes sur la fermentation au laboratoire de Carlsberg. *Revue Scientifique*, Paris: (2nd ser.) 19:851-55.

53. Richet, C. 1880. Les démoniaques d'autrefois. *Revue des Deux Mondes*, Paris: 37:340, 522, 828.

54. Moutard-Martin, R., Richet, C. 1880. De quelques faits relatifs à la sécrétion urinaire. *Comptes rendus de l'Académie des Sciences*, Paris: 80:186-188.

55. Moutard-Martin, R., Richet, C. 1880. Effets des injections intraveinuses du sucre et de gomme. *Comptes rendus de l'Académie des Sciences*, Paris: 90:98.

56. Richet, C. 1880. De quelques faits relatifs à la digestion gastrique des poissons. *Comptes rendus de l'Académie des Sciences*, Paris: 90:879-81.

57. Richet, C. 1880. De l'influence des milieux alcalins ou acides sur la vie des écrevisses. *Comptes rendus de l'Académie des Sciences*, Paris: 17 May, 90:1160.

58. Reynier, P. and C. Richet. 1880. Expériences relatives au choc péritonéal. *Comptes rendus de l'Académie des Sciences*. Paris: 90:1220-23.

59. Richet, C. 1880. De l'action de la strychnine à très forte dose sur les mammifères. *Comptes rendus de l'Académie des Sciences*, Paris: 91:443-45.

60. Richet, C. 1880. De l'onde secondaire du muscle. *Comptes rendus de l'Académie des Sciences*, Paris: 91-828; also *Gazette Médecine de Paris*, (6th ser.) 2:631.

61. Bouchardat, M.G., Richet, C. 1880. Des dérives chlorés et de la strychnine. *Comptes rendus de l'Académie des Sciences*, Paris: 13 Dec. 91:990.

62. Richet C. 1880. D'un mode particulier d'asphyxie dans l'empoisonnement par la strychnine. *Comptes rendus de l'Académie* injections d'urée sur l'elimination de l'urée. *Comptes rendus de l'Académie des Sciences*, Paris: 28 Fev.

63. Richet, C. 1880. Editor of *La Revue Scientifique de la France et de l'étranger*, Paris.

64. Richet, C. 1880. Essai sur les méthodes numériques qui permettent d'apprécier la fécondité et la vitalité. *Review d'Anthropologie* Paris: 103-212.

65. Richet, C. 1880. Observations sur la respiration de quelques poissons marins. *Comptes rendus de la Société de Biologie*, Paris: 30 October, 314-17.

66. Richet, C. 1880. Rapport sur l'organisation des laboratoires de physiologie des Pays-Bas (Amsterdam, Leyden, Utrecht) *Arch. d. Missions Scient.*, 289-300.
67. Richet. C. 1881. The simulation of somnambulism. *Lancet*, London: 1:8-51.
68. Richet, C. 1881. De la rigidité cadavérique. *Revue Scientifique*, Paris: (3d ser.) 1:46-54.
69. Richet, C. 1881. Phénomènes chimiques de la contraction musculaire. *Revue Scientifique*, Paris: (3d ser.) 1:206-15.
70. Richet, C. 1881. Etude historique sur la physiologie du sysème nerveux. *Revue Scientifique*, Paris: (3d ser.) 1:426-33.
71. Richet, C. 1881. A study of the pathological physiology of contractures. *Lancet* 1:815-17.
72. Richet, C. 1881. Sensibilité, nutrition, physiologie pathologique des muscles. *Revue de Médecine*, Paris: 1:1024-43.
73. Richet, C. 1881. De la vibration nerveuse. *Revue Scientifique*, Paris: (3d ser.) 2:98-111.
74. Richet, C. 1881. Des conditions de la vie du cerveau. *Revue Scientifique*, Paris: (3d ser.) 2:801-12.
75. Richet, C. 1881. De la contracture des hystéroépileptiques. *Cong. period. Internat. d. sc. med. Compt. rend. Amst.* 6 (pt. 2) 203.
76. Moutard-Martin, R., Richet, C. 1881. Recherches expérimentales sur la polyurie. *Archives de Physiologie norm. et Pathologie*, Paris: (2nd ser.) 8:1-48.
77. Richet, C. 1881. De l'éxcitabilité réflexe des muscles dans la première période du somnambulisme. *Archives de Physiologie norm. et Pathologie* Paris: (2d ser.) 8:155-57.
78. Richet, C. 1881. De la nutrition; de la coagulation, de la digestion et de la fermentation du lait. *Progrès Médecine*, Paris: 9:175-77; 229-31; 298-316.
79. Richet, C. 1881. De la nutrition; de quelques opinions récentes relatives au suc gastrique. *Progrès Médecine*, Paris: 9:35.
80. Moutard-Martin, R., Richet, C. 1881. Contribution à l'action physiologique de l'urée et des sels ammoniacaux. *Gazette hebd. de Médecine* Paris: (2nd ser.) 18:184.
81. Richet, C. 1881. Des mouvements de la grenouille consécutifs a l'excitation électrique. *Comptes rendus de l'Académie des Sciences*, 92:1298-1301, Paris: also *Archives de Physiologie norm et Pathologie*, (2d ser.) 8:824-37.
82. Richet, C. 1881. De la toxicité comparée des différents métaux. *Comptes rendus de l'Académie des Sciences*, Paris: 93:649-51.
83. Chavanne, A., Richet, C. 1881. Nouveau procédé pour le dosage immédiat des maitières dites extractives de l'urine. *Comptes rendus de la Société de Biologie*, Paris: 30 July, 269-71.
84. Richet, C. 1881. Note relative à la fermentation de l'urée. *Comptes rendus de l'Académie des Sciences*, Paris: 13 March, 730.
85. Moutard-Martin, R., Richet, C. 1881. Effets des injections d'urée sur l'elimination de l'urée. *Comptes rendus de l'Académie des Sciences*, Paris: 28 Fev.
86. Richet, C. 1881. De l'électrisation des ferments. Congrès des sociétés savantes de la Sorbonne. *Revue Scientifique.*, 603.
87. Richet, C. 1881. Du tétanos électrique. *Mémoires lu à l'Académie de médecine dans la séance du.*

88. Richet, C. 1881. Foreword to: Combet, L.: Sarcome primitif des muscles à propos d'un cas observé dans le service de M. le Prof. Richet, Paris: 54.

89. Chavanne, A., Richet, C. 1882. Nouveau procédé pour le dosage immédiat des matières dites extractives de l'urine. *Comptes rendus de la Société de Biologie*, Paris: (7th ser.) 3:269-71.

90. Richet, C. 1882. D l'action tétanisante et paralysante du chlourure de sodium. *Gazette Médecine de Paris* (6th ser.) 4:599-602.

91. Richet, C. 1882. Note sur un nouveau parasite du blé. *Union Médecine et Scientifique*, Du nord-est, Reims 6:265-68.

92. Richet, C. 1882. Action physiologique des metaux alacalins. *Archives de physiologie norm et pathologie*, 9:145-336.

93. Richet, C. 1882. Etude sur 'action physiologique comparée des chlorures alcalins. *Archives de physiologie norm et pathologie* (2nd ser.) 10:145.

94. Richet, C. 1882. De quelques faits relatifs à la digestion chez les poissons. *Archives de physiologie norm. et pathologie* (2nd ser.) 10:536-58.

95. Richet, C. 1882. L'accroissement de la population Française. *Revue des Deux Mondes.* (3d ser.) 50:587-616, 900-32.

96. Rondeau, P. and C. Richet. 1882. Des phénomènes de la mort part le froid chez des mammifères. *Comptes rendus de l'Académie des Sciences*, Paris: 95:931-34; also *Gazette Médecine de Paris* (6th ser.) 4:599-602.

97. Richet, C. 1882. Note sur quelques faits relatifs a l'excitabilité musculaire. *Bulletin de la Société de Biologie*, 21-23.

98. Richet, C. 1882. Reactions chimiques réductrices du lait et de l'urine. *Bulletin de la Société de Biologie*, 233:235, April.

99. Richet, C. 1882. Leçons sur la physiologie générale des muscles, des nerfs et des centres nervueus, 924, Germer Bailliere, (dedicated to Vulpian).

100. Richet, C. 1882. Microbes chez les poissons et les animaux marins. *Bulletin de la Société de Biologie*, 669-72.

101. Rondeau, P., Richet, C. 1882. De la vie des animaux enfermés dans du platre. *Bulletin de la Société de Biologie*, 692-97.

102. Etard, A., Richet, C. 1883. Procédé nouveau dosage des matières extractives et de l'urée. *Archives de Physiologie norm. et Pathologie*, Paris (3d ser.) 1:636-44.

103. Richet, C. 1883. Contribution aux paralyses et aux anesthésies réflexes. *Archives de Physiologie norm. et Pathologie*, Paris (3d ser.) 2:367.

104. Richet, C. 1883. La conversation des fruits par le chloroforme. *Comptes rendus Société de Biologie*, Paris (7th ser.) 4:26.

105. Olivier, L., Richet, C. 1883. Microbes de la lymphe des poissons. *Comptes rendus de l'Académie des Sciences*, Paris: 4:119.

106. Richet, C. 1883. Expériences sur le cerveau des oiseaux. *Comptes rendus Société de Biologie*, Paris (7th ser.) 4:129-133.

107. Richet, C. 1883. Influence de l'acide chlorhydrique sur la fermentation ammonicale de l'urine. *Comptes rendus Société de Biologie*, Paris (7th ser.) 4:436-39.

108. Olivier, L., Richet, C. 1883. Nouvelles expériences sur les microbes de la lymphe des poissons. *Comptes rendus de la Société de Biologie*, Paris (7th ser.) 4:477-80.

109. Richet, C. 1883. Durée des phénomènes reflexes dans l'anémie, chez, les animaux a sang froid. *Comptes rendus Société de Biologie*, Paris (7th ser.) 4:578-581.

110. Richet, C. 1883. Influence de la température sur l'intoxication des poissons. *Comptes rendus Société de Biologie,* Paris (7th ser.) 4:587.
111. Richet, C. 1883. Influence de la pression et de la température sur l'asphyxie des poissons. *Comptes rendus de l'Académie des Sciences,* Paris (7th ser.) 4:584–87.
112. Olivier, L., Richet, C. 1883. Des cristaux de la lymphe des poissons. *Comptes rendus de la Société de Biologie,* Paris; (7th ser.) 4:588.
113. Richet, C. 1883. Hypnotisme et contracture. *Comptes rendus Société,* Paris (7th ser.) 4:662–64.
114. Richet, C. 1883. De diversorum musculorum diversa irritabilitate. *Archives Pflugers Physiology,* Bonn, 31:146.
115. Richet, C. 1883. Deux expériences d'inhibition sur la grenouille et quelques autres faits relatifs à l'inhibition. Paris, 56:1081.
116. Richet, C. 1883. L'étude de la physiologie. *Gazette d'Hôpital Paris,* 56:1081.
117. Olivier, L., Richet, C. 1883. Les microbes des poissons marins. *Comptes rendus de l'Académie des Sciences,* Paris: 96:384 386.
118. Etard, A., Richet, C. 1883. Dosage des matières extractives et du pouvoir réducteur de l'urine. *Comptes rendus de l'Académie des Sciences,* Paris: 96:855–58.
119. Olivier, L., Richet, C. 1883. Nouvelles observations sur les microbes des poissons. *Comptes rendus de l'Académie des Sciences,* Paris: 97:674–77.
120. Richet, C. 1883. De l'action toxique comparée des métaux sur les microbes. *Comptes rendus de l'Académie des Sciences,* Paris 97: 1004–1006.
121. Olivier, L., Richet, C. 1883. Les microbes de la lymphe des poissons marins. *Comptes rendus de l'Académie des Sciences,* Paris: 97:678–84.
122. Richet, C. 1883. La personalite et la mémoire dans le somnabulisme. *Revue Philosophique,* 225–42.
123. Richet, C. 1883. Nouveau procédé de dosage de l'oxygène et de l'acide carbonique de la respiration. *Bulletin de la Société de Biolologie,* 233 and 445, June.
124. Olivier, L., Richet, C. 1883. Des cristaux de la lymphe des poissons. *Bulletin de la Société de Biologie,* 588–594, November 17.
125. Etard, A., Richet, C. 1883. Procédé nouveau de dosage des matières extractives et de l'urée de l'urine. Paris. G. Masson, 636–644.
126. Richet, C. 1883. De la dialyse de l'acide du suc gastrique. *Comptes rendus d l'Académie des Sciences,* Paris, CXVII, 682–85.
127. Richet, C. 1883. La sensibilité gustative pour les metaux. *Bulletin de la Société de Biologie,* 687–90.
128. Richet, C. 1884. Note on mental suggestion. *Brain.* London: 7:83.
129. Richet, C. 1884. Rapport sur un projet de questionnaire d'hérédité psychologique. *Bulletin Sociologie d'Anthropologie de Paris,* (3d ser.) 7:734–40.
130. Richet, C. 1884. L'enseignement de la physiologie à la Faculté de Paris: erreurs et ignorance. "Prog. Méd." (numéro des étudiants); le cours auxiliaire (semestre d'hivere). *Tribune Méd.* Paris: 16:25–28 (continued in next issue 49–55; 3 February, This part was signed by Laborde).
131. Richet, C. 1884. Man's right over animals (Vivisection). *Popular Science Monthly,* New York: 25:759–766; translated from *Revue des Deux Mondes.*
132. Richet, C. 1884. Lavoisier et la Chaleur Animale. *Revue Scientifique,* Paris: 34:141–46.
133. Richet, C. 1884. La température des mammifères et des oiseaux. *Revue Scientifique,* Paris: 34:298–310.

134. Richet, C. 1884. De la dyspnée asphyxique chez le chien. *Comptes rendus de l'Académie des Sciences,* Paris: 99:279–82.

135. Richet, C. 1884. La fièvre traumatique nerveruse et l'influence des lésions du cerveau sur la température général., *Comptes rendus de la Société de Biologie,* 29 March, 189–95, 5 April, 209–16; 19 April, 248–50; also in *Comptes rendus de la Académie des Sciences,* 9 August, 548–56.

136. Richet, C. 1884. L'homme et l'intelligence, fragments de physiologie et de psychologie par Charles Richet . . . Paris: F. Alcan, VII, 570.

137. Richet, C. 1884. Oeuvres de Lavoisier, Lavoisier, A.L.: Mémoire sur la combustion de phospure de Nickel, et sur la nature de l'acide qui résulte de cette combustion. Vol. 2, 139–52.

138. Richet, C. 1884. De la dialyse de l'acide du suc gastrique. *Comptes rendus de l'Académie des Sciences,* Paris: 17 May, 682.

139. Richet, C. 1884. Des diastases chez les poissons. *Comptes rendus de la Société de Biologie,* 16 February, 74–76.

140. Richet, C. 1884. Le calorimètre à siphon et la production de chaleur. *Comptes rendus de la Société de Biologie,* 29 November, 655–715.

141. Pignol, M., Richet, C. 1884. Ferments diastatiques du sang et des tissues. *Comptes rendus de la Société de Biologie,* 23 February, 94–95.

142. Richet, C. 1884. Origine du mot magnétisme animal. *Comptes rendus de la Société de Biologie,* 24 May, 334–35.

143. Richet, C. 1884. Influence de la fréquence de la respiration sur la chaleur chez le chien. *Bulletin de la Société de Biologie,* 9 August, 548–50.

144. Richet, C. 1884. Sur l'emploi des mélanges titrés des vapeurs anesthésiques et d'air dans la chloroformisation. *Comptes rendus de l'Académie des Sciences,* 28 January.

145. Richet, C. 1885. Un fait de somnambulisme à distance. *Bulletin la Société de Psychologie Physiologique,* Paris: 1:33.

146. Richet, C. 1885. La calorimètre par rayonnement. *Comptes rendus de la Société de Biologie,* Paris: (8th ser.) 2:2–8.

147. Gley, E., Richet, C. 1885. Dosage de l'azote total de l'urine par l'hypobromite de sodium titré. *Comptes rendus de l'Académie des Sciences,* Paris: (8th ser.) 2:136–38.

148. Richet, C. 1885. L'élimination des boissons par l'urine. *Comptes rendus de la Société de Biologie,* Paris: (8th ser.) 2:563–66.

149. Gley, E., Richet, C. 1885. Action chimique et sensibilité gustative. *Comptes rendus Société de Biologie,* Paris: (8th ser.) 2:742–46.

150. Richet, C. 1885. Recherches de calorimètre. *Archives de Physiologie norm. et Pathologie* Paris: (3d ser.) 6:237–91; 450–97.

151. Richet, C. 1885. Leçons sur la chaleur animale. La température des animaux à sang froid. *Revue Scientifique,* Paris: 35:202–12.

152. Richet, C. 1885. La température normale de l'homme. *Revue Scientifique,* Paris: 35:424–34; 620–29.

153. Richet, C. 1885. La température du corps des malades. *Revue Scientifique,* Paris: 36:295–306.

154. Richet, C. 1885. Leçons sur la chaleur animale; la température apres la mort. *Revue Scientifique,* Paris: 36:398–403.

155. Richet, C. 1885. Les muscles et la production de la Chaleur. *Revue Scientifique,* Paris: 36:488–97.

156. Richet, C. 1885. Les muscles et la production de la chaleur. *Revue Scientifique,* Paris: 36:488-97.
157. Richet, C. 1885. Die Beziehungen des Gehirns zur Körperwärme und zum Fieberg. *Archives Pflugers Physiology,* Bonn: 37:624.
158. Richet, C. 1885. Influence du système nerveux sur la calorification. *Comptes rendus de l'Académie des Sciences,* Paris: 100:1021-24.
159. Richet, C. 1885. Observations calorimétrique sur les enfants. *Comptes rendus de l'Académie des Sciences,* Paris: 100:1602-04.
160. Richet, C. 1885. De l'action physiologique des sels de lithium, de potassium et de rubidium. *Comptes rendus de l'Académie des Sciences,* Paris: 101:667; 707-10.
161. Gley, M. M., Richet, C. 1885. Action chimique et sensibilité gustative. *Comptes rendus de la Société de Biologie,* Paris: 742.
162. Richet, C. 1885. *Essai de Psychologie Générale.* Paris: F. Alcan.
163. Gley, M. M., Richet, C. 1885. Dosage de l'azote total de l'urine par l'hypobromite de sodium titré. *Comptes rendus de la Société de Biologie,* 563-66.
164. Richet, C. 1885. De quelques températures élèves auxquelles peuvent vivre des animaux marins. *Archives de Zoologie Expérimentale.*
165. Richet, C. 1885. Recherches de calorimetre. *Archives de Physiologie,* 237-58, 450-97.
166. Gley, M. M., Richet, C, 1885. Expériences sur la haschisch. *Bulletin de la Société de Psychologie Physiologique,* 9-13.
167. Richet, C. 1885. Influence de la cocaine et du chloroforme sur la production de la chaleur. *Comptes rendus de la Société de Biologie,* 11 January, 8-10.
168. Richet, C. 1885. De la calorimétre. *Comptes rendus de la Société de Biologie,* 6 February, 98-99.
169. Richet, C. 1885. L'action toxique suivant la température. *Comptes rendus de la Société de Biologie,* 18 April, 239-41.
170. Richet, C. 1885. La sensibilité gustative pour les alcaloides. *Comptes rendus de la Société de Biologie,* 18 June, 377-85.
171. Richet, C. 1885. Hyperthermie consecutive aux lesions du cerveau. *Comptes rendus de la Société de Biologie,* 26 June, 304-6.
172. Richet, C. 1885. Observations calorimétriques chez les enfants. *Comptes rendus de l'Académie des Sciences,* 29 June, 1602.
173. Richet, C. 1885. Effets de l'éxcitation tramatique du cerveau chez les lapins. *Comptes rendus de la Société de Biologie,* 18 July, 487-89.
174. Richet, C. 1885. Milieux acides ou basiques dans lesquels peuvent vivre les poissons de mer. *Comptes rendus de la Société de Biologie,* 6 November, 482-88.
175. Gley, E., Richet, C., Rondeau, P. 1886. Notes sur le haschisch. *Bulletin Société de Psychologie Physiologique,* Paris: 1:9-13.
176. Richet, C. 1886. Des rapports de l'hallucination avec l'état mental. *Bull. Société de Psychologie Physiologique,* Paris: 1:21-23.
177. Richet, C. 1886. Un fait de somnambulisme à distance. *Bulletin Société de Psychologie Physiologique,* Paris: 1:33.
178. Richet, C. 1886. De l'hyperthermie consécutive aux lesions du cerveau. *Comptes rendus de la Société de Biologie,* Paris: (8th ser.) 3:304-6.
179. Richet, C. 1886. Expériences sur le cerveau des oiseaux. *Comptes rendus de la Société de Biologie,* Paris: (8th ser.) 3:306.
180. Richet, C., Co-editor. 1886-1887. *Archives slaves de Biologie.* Paris.

181. Richet, C. 1886. Influence de la fréquence de la respiration sur la chaleur chez le chien. *Comptes rendus de la Société de Biologie*, Paris (8th ser.) 3:397-99.

182. Richet, C. 1886. Expériences sur la vie des poissons dans divers milieux et sur l'action physiologique des differents sels de soude. *Comptes rendus de la Société de Biologie*, Paris: (8th ser.) 3:482-89.

183. Hanriot, M., Richet, C. 1886. Nouveau procédé de dosage de l'oxygène et de l'acide carbonique de la respiration. *Comptes rendus de la Société de Biologie*, Paris (8th ser.) 3:621.

184. Richet, C. 1886. Du coéfficient de dénutrition. *Comptes rendus de la Société de Biologie*, Paris: (8th ser.) 3:623-27.

185. Richet, C. 1886. De l'action physiologique des sels alcalins; études de toxicologie générale. *Archives de Physiologie norm. et Pathologie*, Paris: (3d ser.) 7:101-50.

186. Mendelssohn, M., Richet, C. 1886. Revue des travaux slaves de physiologie pour l'année. *Archives Slaves de Biology*, Paris: 8:71.

187. Richet, C. 1886. La peur; étude psychologique. *Revue des Deux Mondes*, Paris: 76:73-117; transl. *Popular Science Monthly*, New York: 29:771-84.

188. Richet, C. 1886. De l'action toxique des sels alcalins. *Comptes rendus de l'Académie des Sciences*, Paris: 102:57-60.

189. Richet, C. 1886. Le travail psychique et la force chimique. *Revue Scientifique*, Paris: 38-788.

190. Richet, C. 1886. Les mouvements inconscients. In *Hommage à M. Chevreul, à l'occasion de son centenaire*. Paris: F. Alcan, 79-94.

191. Ferrari, M. M. H., Héricourt, J., Richet, C. 1886. La personnalité et l'écriture. *Bulletin de la Société de Psychologie Physiologique*, 21-30.

192. Richet, C. 1886. La pensée et le travail chimique. *Revue Scientifique*, Paris: 83.

193. Richet, C. 1886. De l'action physiologique de sels alcalins; études de toxicologie générale. Paris: G. Masson, 101-150. Cutting from *Archives de Physiologie norm. et Pathologie*, 7, (3d ser.) Paris.

194. Richet, C. 1886. A propos des jeûneurs. *Gaz. hebd. de méd. et de chir.*, 854.

195. Richet, C. 1886. Action physiologique des métaux alcalin. *Archives de Physiologie norm. et Pathologie*, 180.

196. Hanriot, M., Richet, C. 1886. Des échanges respiratoire chez l'homme, *Comptes rendus de la Société de Biologie*, 39, 621.

197. Richet, C. 1886. Expériences sur le reflexe de direction de l'oreille chez le lapin. *Comptes rendus de la Société de Biologie*, Paris: (8th ser.) 19 June, 3:307.

198. Richet, C. 1887. Effets de l'hypnotisme sur l'insomnie *Comptes rendus de la Société de Biologie*, Paris: (8th ser.) 4:35.

199. Gley, E., Richet, C. 1887. Expériences sur la courbe horaire de l'urée et le dosage de l'azoté total de l'urine. *Comptes rendus de la Société de Biologie*, Paris: (8th ser.) 4:377-85.

200. Hanriot, M., Richet, C. 1887. De l'élimination de l'acide carbonique dans les injections rectales de ce gas. *Comptes rendus de la Société de Biologie*, Paris: (8th ser.) 4:405.

201. Richet, C. 1887. Régulation de la température chez le chien. *Comptes rendus de la Société de Biologie*, Paris: (8th ser.) 4:482-84.

202. Hanriot, M., Richet, C. 1887. Note sur l'absorption le l'acide carbonique et sur l'inscription graphique de l'acide carbonique exhale. *Comptes rendus de la Société de Biologie*, Paris: (8th ser.) 4:753.

203. Richet, C. 1887. Dosage de l'acide carbonique expiré après lavement gazeux d'acide carbonique. *Comptes rendus de la Société Physiologie et de Psychologie*, (2d ed), Paris: F. Alcan, 570.

204. Richet, C. 1887. L'homme et l'intelligence. Fragments de physiologie et de psychologe, (2nd ed.): Paris: F. Alcan, 5-570.

205. Richet, C. 1887. Expériences sur le poids des animaux. *Archives de physiologie norm. et Pathologie*, (3d ser.) 10:473-94.

206. Richet, C. 1887. De la composition typographique et du style de quelques livres imprimés. *Revue Philosophique*, Paris: 23:108-12.

207. Richet, C. 1887. L'instinct. *Revue Scientifique*, Paris: 39:648-58.

208. Richet, C. 1887. Le système nerveux et la chaleur animale. *Revue Scientifique*, Paris: 40:353-60.

209. Richet, C. 1887. La regulation de la chaleur par la respiration. *Revue Scientifique*, Paris: 40:513-19.

210. Richet, C. 1887. La circulation capillaire et la chaleur animale. (Reponse à de R. de Latour). *Revue Scientifique*, Paris: 40:564.

211. Richet, C. 1887. Leçons sur la chaleur animale; la respiration et la température. *Revue Scientifique*, Paris: 40:801-11.

212. Hanriot, M., Richet, C. 1887. Nouveau procédé de dosage de l'acide carbonique expiré et de l'oxygène absorbé dans les actes respiratoires. *Comptes rendus de l'Académie des Sciences*, Paris:104:435-37.

213. Hanriot, M., Richet, C. 1887. Relations du travail musculaire avec les actions chimiques respiratoires. *Comptes rendus de l'Académie des Sciences*, 105:76-79.

214. Hanriot, M., Richet, C. 1887. Influence des modifications volontaires de la respiration sur l'excrétion de l'acide carbonique. *Comptes rendus de l'Académie des Sciences*. Paris: 104:1327-30.

215. Hanriot, M., Richet, C. 1887. Influence du travail musculaire sur le échanges respiratoires. *Comptes rendus de l'Académie des Sciences*. Paris: 1904:1865-69.

216. Richet, C. 1887. Des conditions de la polypnée thermique. *Comptes rendus de l'Académie des Sciences*, Paris: 105:313-16.

217. Richet, C. 1887. De quelques conditions qui modifient le rythme respiratoire. *Comptes rendus de la Société de Biologie*, Paris: (8th ser.) 4 (pt.2): 24-35.

218. Richet, C. 1887. Influence de la fréquence de la respiration sur la chaleur chez le chien. *Comptes rendus de la Société de Biologie*, 25-35.

219. Richet, C. 1887. La physiologie et la médecine. Leçon inaugurale du cours de physiologie de la faculté de médecine, *Revue Scientifique*. Paris.

220. Richet, C. 1887. Possession, par Charles Epheyre (2nd ed.). Paris: Ollendorf, 275.

221. Hanriot, M., Richet, C. 1887. Présentation d'un Spiromètre. *Comptes rendus de la Société de Biologie*, Paris: (8th ser.).

222. Richet, C. 1887-1888. Expériences sur le sommeil à distance. *Revue de l'Hypnotique Experimentale et Therapie*, Paris: 2:225-40.

223. Richet, C. 1888. Nouvelle fonction du bulbe rachidien; régulation de la température par la respiration. *Archives de Physiologie norm. et Pathologie*, Paris: (4th ser.) 1:193-211, 292.

224. Baillière, P., Richet, C. 1888. Expérience sur la mort par hyperthermie. *Comptes rendus de la Société de Biologie*, Paris: (8th ser.) 5:417.

225. Hanriot, M., Richet, C. 1888. Des phénomènes chimiques de la respiration dans le tétanos électrique. *Comptes rendus de la Société de Biologie*, Paris (8th ser.) 5:75-81.

226. Richet, C. 1888. Les reflexes psychiques. *Revue Philosophique*, Paris: 25:225, 387, 500.

227. Richet, C. 1888. La physiologie et la médecine. *Revue Scientifique*, Paris: 41:353, 426.

228. Hanriot, M., Richet, C. 1888. Influence des différents alimenations sur le échanges gazeux respiratoires. *Comptes rendus de l'Académie des Sciences*, Paris: 106:496-98.

229. Langlois, P., Richet, C. 1888. Influence de la température organique sur les convulsions de la cocaine *Comptes rendus de l'Académie des Sciences*,Paris: 106:1616-18.

230. Héricourt, J., Richet, C. 1888. Sur un microbe pyogène et septique (staphylococcus pyosepticus) et sur la vaccination contre ses éffets. *Comptes rendus de l'Académie des Sciences*, Paris: 107:690-92.

231. Héricourt, J., Richet, C. 1888. De la transfusion péritonéale et de l'immunité qu'elle confére. *Comptes rendus de l'Académie des Sciences*, Paris: 107:748-50; also, *France Médecine* Paris: 2:1604-6.

232. Richet, C. 1888. Durée des phénomènes reflexes dans l'anémie, chez les animaux à sang froid. *Comptes rendus de la Société de Biologie*, 10 November, 578-81.

233. Richet, C. 1888. Du poids relatif des divers organes chez les poissons. *Comptes rendus de la Société de Biologie*, 24 November, 780-82.

234. Richet, C. 1888. Notes de technique de physiologie. 1. Injections péritonéals pour l'anesthesie. 2. Disposition de la soupage de Muller pour la respiration spontanée et la respiration artificielle. 3. Procédé pour conserver longtemps du sang frais sans altérations et sans sterilisation. 4. Action des vapeurs de mercure. *Comptes rendus de la Société de Biologie*, 21 December, 727-31.

235. Richet, C. 1888. Influence de l'alimentation chez l'homme sur la fixation et l'élimination de carbone. *Comptes rendus de l'Académie des Sciences*, Paris: 6 February, 419.

236. Langlois, J. P., Richet, C. 1888. Influence du chloral sur la force des centres nerveux respiratoires. *Comptes rendus de la Société de Biologie*, 779-80.

237. Richet, C. 1888. La physiologie et la médecine leçon d'ouverture de cours de physiologie de la Faculté de Médecine de Paris, Par. M. Charles Richet, Paris: Maison Quantin.

238. Héricourt, J., Richet, C. 1889. Influence de la transfusion péritonéale du sang de chien sur l'évolution de la tuberculose chez le lapin. *Comptes rendus de la Société de Biologie*, Paris: (9th ser.) 1:157-63.

239. Langlois, J. P., Richet, C. 1889. Influence de la température organique sur les convulsions. *Archives de Physiologie norm. et Pathologie*, Paris: (5th ser.) 1:181-96.

240. Langlois, J. P., Richet, C. 1889. De la ventilation pulmonaire. *Comptes rendus de la Société de Biologie*, Paris: (9th ser.) 1:304.

241. Richet, C. 1889. Notes de technique physiologique. *Comptes rendus de la Société de Biologie*, Paris: (9th ser.) 1:727-31.

242. Richet, C. 1889. L'inanition chez les animaux. *Revue Scientifique*, Paris: 43:641, 711.
243. Richet, C. 1889. Le génie et la folie. *Revue Scientifique*, Paris: 42:795–800; 43:83–85.
244. Richet, C. 1889. L'inanition chez l'homme. *Revue Scientifique*, Paris: 43:801; 44:106.
245. Richet, C. 1889. Le jeûne chez l'homme. *Revue Scientifique*, 44:106.
246. Richet, C. 1889. Le jeûne chez les animaux. *Revue Scientifique*, 44:641.
247. Héricourt, J., Richet, C. 1889. De la transfusion péritonéale et de la toxicité variable du sang de chien pour les lapin. *Comptes rendus de l'Académie des Sciences*, Paris: 108:623–25.
248. Langlois, J. P., Richet, C. 1889. Influence des anesthésiques sur la force des mouvements respiratoires. *Comptes rendus de l'Académie des Sciences*, Paris: 108:681–83.
249. Richet, C. 1889. Régulation, par le système nerveux des combustions respiratoires, en rapport avec la taille de l'animal. *Comptes rendus de l'Académie des Sciences*, Paris: 109:190–92.
250. Richet, C. 1889. Influence de la transfusion peritonéale du sang de chien sur l'évolution de la tuberculose chez le lapin. *Comptes rendus de la Société de Biologie*, 2 March, 157–163.
251. Héricourt, J., Richet, C. 1889. Sur un microbe pyogène et septique et sur la vaccination contre ses effets. *Arch. de Médecine Expérimentale*, 674–95.
252. Richet, C. 1889. Influence de anesthésiques sur la force des mouvements respiratoires. *Comptes rendus de l'Académie des Sciences*, April, 681.
253. Richet, C. 1889. De la ventilation pulmonaire. *Comptes rendus de la Société de Biologie*, 20 April, 304–5.
254. Richet, C. 1889. Cécité psychique expérimentale chez le chien. *Congress Internationale de Psychologie Physiologie de 1889*, Séance du. 8 August, 63–65.
255. Richet, C. 1889. Foreword to: Lombroso, C.: L'homme de génie. *Trad. sur la 6th ed. Italienne par F.C. d'Istria et precédé d'une.* Préface de C. Richet. Paris: F. Alcan, 499.
256. Richet, C. 1889. La Chaleur Animale, Paris: F. Alcan.
257. Richet, C. 1889. Nouveau procédé d'anesthésie pour les animaux. *Comptes rendus de la Société de Biologie*, (9th ser.) 21 December.
258. Héricourt, J., Richet, C. 1890. Effets de l'infusion du sang de chien à des lapins sur l'évolution de la tuberculose. *Comptes rendus de la Société de Biologie*, Paris: (9th ser.) 1:316, 325.
259. Richet, C. 1890. Mesure des combustions respiratoires, chez le chien. *Archives de Physiologie norm. et Pathologie*, Paris: (5th ser.) 2:17–30.
260. Richet, C. 1890. De l'influence du chloral sur les actions chimiques respiratoires chez le chien. *Archives de Physiology norm. et Pathologie* Paris: (5th ser.) 2:221–31.
261. Langlois, J. P., Richet, C. 1890. Troubles trophiques bilatéraux après lésions de l'écorce cérébrale. *Comptes rendus de la Société de Biologie*, Paris: (9th ser.) 2:315.
262. Richet, C. 1890. De la mesure des combustions respiratoires chez les oiseaux. *Archives de Physiologie norm. et Pathologie*, Paris: (5th ser.) 2:483–95.
263. Héricourt, J., Richet, C. 1890. Expériences sur la vaccination anti-tuberculeuse. *Comptes rendus de la Société de Biologie*, Paris: (9th ser.) 2:627–30.

264. Héricourt, J., Richet, C. 1890. De l'immunité contre la tuberculose par les transfusions de sang chien tuberculeux. *Comptes rendus de la Société de Biologie*, Paris: 3:630-33.

265. Richet, C. 1889-1890. Further experiments in hypnotic lucidity or clairvoyance (transl.). *Procédé Sociologie Psychologie Research*, London: 6:66-83.

266. Richet, C. 1890. Action du sulfate de quinine contre le mal de mer. *Progrès Médecine* Paris (2nd ser.) 12:190.

267. Richet, C. 1890. Les hallucinations télépathiques. *Revue Scientifique*, Paris: 46:784-87.

268. Richet, C. 1890. Le rythme de la respiration. *Revue Scientifique*, Paris: 46:788-91.

269. Héricourt, J., Richet, C. 1890. Influence de la transfusion péritonéale du sang de chien sur l'évolution de la tuberculose chez le lapin. *Comptes rendus de l'Académie des Sciences*, Paris: 110:1282-84.

270. Héricourt, J., Richet, C. 1890. De l'action toxique des extraits alcooliques du sang et des divers tissues. *Comptes rendus de la Société de Biologie*, 13 December, 695.

271. Richet, C. 1890. De l'immunité conferée à des lapins par la transfusion péritonéale du sang de chien. Etudes sur la tuberculose. *Comptes rendus de la Société de Biologie*, 380-411, 678-80.

272. Richet, C. 1890. De la vaccination contre la tuberculose par produits solubles des cultures tuberculeuses. Etudes sur la tuberculose. *Comptes rendus de la Société de Biologie*, 15 November, 1-15, 627-30.

273. Langlois, J. P., Richet, C. 1890. De la sensibilité musculaire de la respiration. *Comptes rendus de la Société de Psychologie Physiologie*, 8-12.

274. Richet, C. 1890. L'homme et l'intelligence. Fragments de physiologie et de psychologie. (2d ed) Paris: F. Alcan.

275. Richet, C. 1890. Foreword to: Manasenia, M.M.: Le surménage mental dans la civilization moderne, èffets, causes remèdes. Traduit du russe par E. Jaubert avec un préface par Charles Richet, Paris: Masson, 286.

276. Richet, C. 1890. La douleur des autres. Paris: Ollendorf.

277. Langlois, J. P. and C. Richet. 1891. Influence des pressions extérieures sur la ventilation pulmonaire. *Archives de Physiologie norm. et Pathologie*, Paris: (5th ser.) 3:1-19.

278. Héricourt, J., Richet, C. 1891. Technique des procédés pour obtenir du serum par de chien et l'innocuité des injections de ce liquide chez l'homme. *Comptes rendus de la Société de Biologie*, Paris: (9th ser.) 3:33-35.

279. Richet, C. 1891. Influence de l'altitude sur l'anémie cérébrale. *Comptes rendus Société de Biologie*, Paris: (9th ser.) 3:35.

280. Héricourt, J., Richet, C. 1891. Nouvelles observations sur la transfusion du sang de chien pour obtenir l'immunité contre la tuberculose. Etudes expér. et clin. s. la tuberculose (Verneuil et al) Paris: 3:139-45.

281. Héricourt, J., Richet, C. 1891. Nouvelles expériences sur les effets des injections de serum dans la tuberculose. *Comptes rendus de la Société de Biologie*, Paris (9th ser.) 3:335-45.

282. Richet, C. 1891. De la mesure des combustions respiratoires chez les mammifères. *Archives de Physiologie norm. et Pathologie* (5th ser.) 3:74-86.

283. Héricourt, J., Richet, C. 1891. De la toxicité des substances solubles des cultures tuberculeuses. *Comptes rendus de la Société de Biologie*, Paris: (9th ser.) 3:470-72.

284. Richet, C. 1891. De la toxicité des sels minéraux (bromures, iodures et chlorures). *Comptes rendus Société de Biologie*, Paris: (9th ser.) 3:744.

285. Héricourt, J., Richet, C. 1891. Pathologie expérimentale de la toxicité des substances solubles des cultures tuberculeuses. *Gazette Médecine de Paris*, (7th ser.) 8:349.

286. Héricourt, J., Richet, C. 1891. De l'état réfractaire du singe à la tuberculose aviaire. *Comptes rendus Société de Biologie*, Paris: (9th ser.) 3:802–804; also *Gazette Médecine de Paris*, (7th ser.) 8:617.

287. Héricourt, J., Richet, C. 1891. Pathologie expérimentale de la toxicité des substances solubles de cultures tuberculeuses. *Gazette Médecine de Paris* (7th ser.) 8:349.

288. Hanriot, M., Richet, C. 1891. Des échanges respiratoires chez l'homme. *Ann de chim*. Paris (6th ser.) 22:495–559.

289. Richet, C. 1891. Qu'est-ce que la physiologie générale? *Revue Scientifique*, Paris: 31:387–97.

290. Richet, C. 1891. L'accroissement de la population Française. *Revue Scientifique*, Paris: 47:518–26.

291. Héricourt, J., Richet, C. 1891. De la toxicité des produits solubles des cultures tuberculeuses. *Comptes rendus de l'Académie des Sciences*, Paris: 112:589–91.

292. Richet, C. 1891. Experimentelle Studien auf dem Gebiete der Gedankenubertragung und des sogenannten Hellsehens. Autorisierte Deutsche Ausgabe von Albert Freiherrn von Schrenk-Notzing. Stuttgart: F. Enke, 254.

293. Héricourt, J., Richet, C. 1891. De la vaccination contre la tuberculose par produits solubles des cultures tuberculeuses. Etudes exper. et clin. s. la tuberculose (Verneuil et al) Paris: 124–38.

294. Richet, C. 1891. Pour les grands et les petits. fables. Préface de M. Sully-Prudhomme. Paris: Libraires-imprimeries réunies, 67.

295. Richet, C. 1891. Cours de physiologie. Programme sommaire. *Bureaux des Revues*, Paris: 350.

296. Richet, C. 1891. Foreword to Gurney, E., Myers, F.W.H. and F. Podmore. Les hallucinations télépathiques; traduit et abrégé des "Phantasms of the Living," par L. Marillier, avec une préface de Charles Richet, Paris: F. Alcan, 395.

297. Richet, C. 1891. Essai de psychologie générale. Paris: (2d ed)., F. Alcan, 176.

298. Richet, C. 1891. Foreword to: Ochorowicz, J.: Mental suggestion, with a preface by Charles Richet. Transl. from the French by J. Fitzgerald, New York, 369.

299. Richet, C. 1891. Cours de physiologie. Programme sommaire. *Bureaux des Revues*, Paris: 350.

300. Hanriot, M., Richet, C. 1891. Des effets physiologiques et toxiques du nickel carbonyl (Ni[CO]4). *Comptes rendus de la Société de Biologie*, 14 March, 185–87.

301. Héricourt, J., Richet, C. 1892. La vaccination tuberculeuse chez le chien. *Gazette Médecine de Paris*, (8th ser.) 1:512.

302. Richet, C. 1892. De la résistance du singe à l'empoisonnement par l'atropine. *Comptes rendus de la Société de Biologie*, Paris: (9th ser.) 4:238.

303. Héricourt, J., Richet, C. 1892. De l'introduction de la rate de chien dans le péritoine des lapins. *Archives de Physiologie norm. et pathologie*. Paris: (5th ser.) 4:597.

304. Richet, C. 1892. Le frisson comme appareil de regulation thermique. *Comptes rendus de la Société de Biologie*, Paris: (9th ser.) 4:896–99.

305. Héricourt, J., Richet, C. 1892. Note sur les effets de la tuberculose aviaire; vaccinant contre la tuberculose humaine chez les singes et les chiens. *Comptes rendus de la*

Société de Biologie, Paris: (9th ser.) 5:58–60; also *Comptes rendus de l'Académie des Sciences*, 116:854.

306. Richet, C. 1892. L'alimentation et le luxe; réponse a L. Tolstoi. *Revue Scientifique*, Paris: 50:385–91.

307. Héricourt, J., Richet, C. 1892. La vaccination tuberculeuse sur le chien. *Comptes rendus de l'Académie des Sciences*, Paris: 114:854–57, 1389–92.

308. Richet, C. 1892. De l'action de quelques sels métalliques sur la fermentation lactique. *Comptes rendus de l'Académie des Sciences*, Paris: 114:1494–1596.

309. Héricourt, J., Richet, C. 1892. Influence sur l'infection tuberculeuse de la transfusion du sang des chiens vaccinés contre la tuberculose. *Compte rendus de l'Académie des Sciences*, Paris: 115:842.

310. Richet, C. 1892. Innocuité de la tuberculose aviaire chez le singe. *Comptes rendus de la Société de Biologie*, 5 November, 846–47.

311. Richet, C. 1892. Effets de la tuberculose aviaire, vaccinant contre la tuberculose humaine chez le singes et les chiens. *Comptes rendus de la Société de Biologie*, January, 58–61.

312. Richet, C. 1892. Des lésions cérébrales dans la cécité psychique expérimentale chez le chien. *Comptes rendus de la Société de Biologie*, 20 February and 19 March, 146–48.

313. Richet, C. 1892. De la vaccination contre la tuberculose humaine par la tuberculose aviaire. Etudes sur la tuberculose, 365–89.

314. Richet, C. 1892. Dans Cent Ans, 2nd ed., Paris: Ollendorf, 295.

315. Langlois, J. P., Richet, C. 1892. Note sur les récents travaux de calorimétre. Travaux de Laboratoire de Ch. Richet, 342.

316. Richet, C. 1892. Bibliothèque Retrospective. Victor Albrecht Von Haller 1708–1777. Mémoire sur la sensibilité - Réponse a quelques objections. Paris: G. Masson.

317. Richet, C. 1892. Bibliothèque Retrospective. Marie François Xavier Bichat. L'influence que la mort du poumon exerce sur la mort du coeur. Paris: Masson.

318. Richet, C. 1893. Contribution à la physiologie des centres nerveux et des muscles de l'écrevisse. *Physiologie Travaux du Laboratoire* Paris: 1:1–93.

319. Richet, C. 1893. De mouvements de la grenouille consécutifs à l'excitation électrique. *Physiologie Travaux du Laboratoire*, Paris: 1:94–108.

320. Hanriot, M., Richet, C. 1893. De l'action physiologique du parachloralose. *Comptes rendus Société de Biologie*, 1:109–29.

321. Langlois, J. P., Richet, C. 1893. De la sensibilité musculaire de la respiration. *Physiologie Travaux du Laboratoire*, Paris: F. Alcan, 1:135–38.

322. Richet, C. 1893. Durée des phénomènes reflexes dans l'anémie chez les animaux à sang froid. *Physiologie Travaux du Laboratoire*, Paris: 1:139–42.

323. Richet, C. 1893. Deux expériences d'inhibition sur la grenouille et quelques autres faits relatifs à inhibition. *Physiologie Travaux du Laboratoire*, Paris: 1:143–46.

324. Richet, C. 1893. Recherches de calorimetre. *Physiologie Travaux du Laboratoire*, Paris: 1:147–255.

325. Richet, C. 1893. Expériences sur le poids des animuax. *Physiologie Travaux du Laboratoire*, Paris: 1:256–73.

326. Langlois, J. P., Richet, C. 1893. Contribution à l'étude de la calorimetre chez l'homme. *Physiology Travaux du Laboratoire*, Paris: 1:279–352.

327. Hanriot, M., Richet, C. 1893. Des échanges respiratoires chez l'homme. *Physiologie Travaux du Laboratoire*, Paris: 1:470-531.

328. Langlois, J. P., Richet, C. 1893. Mesure des combustions respiratoires chez le chien. *Physiology Travaux du Laboratoire*, Paris: F. Alcan, 1:532-47.

329. Langlois, J. P., Richet, C. 1893. De l'influence du chloral sur les actions chimiques respiratoires chez le chien. *Physiology Travaux du Laboratoire*, Paris: F. Alcan, 1:548-59.

330. Richet, C.: 1893. La physiologie et la médecine. *Physiologie Travaux du Laboratoire*, Paris: 2:1-54.

331. Richet, C. 1893. Notes de technique physiologique. *Physiologie Travaux du Laboratoire*, Paris: 2:175-80.

332. Moutard-Martin, R., Richet, C. 1893. Recherches expérimentale sur la polyurie. *Physiologie Travaux du Laboratoire*, Paris: F. Alcan, 2:181-233.

333. Richet, C. 1893. Influence de la pression et de la température sur l'asphyxie des poissons. *Physiologie Travaux du Laboratoire*, Paris: 2:260-63.

334. Richet, C. 1893. L'inanition. *Physiologie Travaux du Laboratoire*, Paris: 2:267-325.

335. Rondeau, P., Richet, C. 1893. Sur la vie des animaux enfermés dans du platre. *Physiologie Travaux du Laboratoire*, Paris: F. Alcan, 2:326-32.

336. Langlois, J. P., Richet, C. 1893. Influence des pressions extérieures sur la ventilation pulmonaire. *Physiologie Travaux du Laboratoire*, Paris: F. Alcan, 2:333-51.

337. Etard, A., Richet, C. 1893. Procédé nouveau de dosage des matières extractives et de l'urée de l'urine. *Physiologie Travaux du Laboratoire*, Paris: F. Alcan, 2:352-63.

338. Richet, C. 1893. L'élimination des boissons par l'urine. *Physiologie Travaux du Laboratoire*, Paris: 2:364-68.

339. Gley, E., Richet, C. 1893. Dosage de l'azote total de l'urine par l'hypobromite de sodium. *Physiologie Travaux du Laboratoire*, Paris: F. Alcan, 2:369-80.

340. Richet, C. 1893. Poids du cerveau, de la rate et du foie chez les chiens de différents tailles. *Physiologie Travaux du Laboratoire*, Paris: 2:381-97.

341. Richet, C. 1893. Action physiologique comparée des métaux alcalins. *Physiologie Travaux du Laboratoire*, Paris: 2:398-441.

342. Gley, E., Richet, C. 1893. De la sensibilitè gustative aux alcaloides. *Physiologie Travaux du Laboratoire*, Paris: F. Alcan, 2:494-96.

343. Richet, C. 1893. Quelques faits relatifs à la digestion chez les poissons. *Physiologie Travaux du Laboratoire*, Paris: 2:536-58.

344. Richet, C. 1893. Expériences de Milan. *Ann. d. sc. psych.*, Paris: 3:1-31.

345. Richet, C. 1893. Des phénomènes chimiques du frisson. *Comptes rendus de la Société de Biologie*, Paris (9th ser.) 5:33-35.

346. Hanriot, M., Richet, C. 1893. Effets physiologiques du chloralose. *Comptes rendus de la Société de Biologie*, Paris: (9th ser.) 5:109, 129 (pt. 2).

347. Héricourt, J., Richet, C. 1893. De quelques expériences relatives à la proportion relative des leucocytes et des hématies dans le sang du chien. *Comptes rendus de la Société de Biologie*, Paris (9th ser.) 5:187-192 (pt. 2).

348. Héricourt, J., Richet, C. 1893. Vaccination du singe contre la tuberculose. *Comptes rendus de la Société de Biologie*, Paris (9th ser.) 5:238-41.

349. Richet, C. 1893. Le frisson comme appareil de regulation thermique. *Gazette Médecine de Paris*, (8th ser.) 5:312-326.

350. Héricourt, J., Richet, C. 1893. Deux expériences sur la tuberculose expérimentale chez le chien. *Comptes rendus de la Société de Biologie*, Paris: (9th ser.) 5:413-15.

351. Richet, C. 1893. Notes sur le rapport entre la toxicité et les propriétés physiques des corps. *Comptes rendus de la Société de Biologie*, Paris: (9th ser.) 5:775.

352. Héricourt, J., Richet, C. 1893. Modifications dans le nombre des leucocytes du sang après injections de diverses substances. *Comptes rendus de la Société de Biologie*, Paris: (9th ser.) 5:965-69.

353. Richet, C. 1893. Un nouvel hypnotique; le chloralose. *Revue Scientifique*, Paris: 51:175-78.

354. Richet, C. 1893. Les procédés de défense de l'organisme. *Revue Scientifique*, Paris: 52:801-7.

355. Hanriot, M., Richet, C. 1893. D'une substance dérivée du chloral ou chloralose et de ses effets physiologiques et thérapéutiques. *Comptes rendus de l'Académie des Sciences*, Paris: 116:63-65.

356. Chassevant, A., Richet, C. 1893. De l'influence des poisons minéraux su la fermentation lactique. *Comptes rendus de l'Académie des Sciences*, Paris: 117:673-75.

357. Richet, C. 1893. Des diastases chez les poissons. *Physiologie Travaux du Laboratoire*, Paris: 264-66.

358. Richet, C. 1893. Le frisson comme appareil de régulation thermique. *Archives de Physiologie*, 312-26.

359. Richet, C. 1893. Effets psychiques du chloralose sur les animaux. *Comptes rendus de la Société de Biologie*, 28 January, 129-31.

360. Richet, C. 1893. De l'action physiologique du parachloralose. *Comptes rendus de la Société de Biologie*, 10 June, (9 ser.) 614-15.

361. Richet, C. 1893. Rapport entre la toxicité et les propriétés des corps. *Comptes rendus de la Société de Biologie*, 22 July, 775-76.

362. Hanriot, M., Richet, C. 1893. De l'action physiologique du chloralose. *Biologie, Mémoires*, 1-7.

363. Richet, C.: 1893. Foreword to Langlois, J.P. and de Varigny, H. Eléments nouveaux de physiologie, précédés d'une introduction par Charles Richet. Paris: O. Doin, 946.

364. Richet, C. 1893. Tuberculose expérimentale du chien. Influence de la dose et des substances solubles. *Congrès de la Tuberculose*, 263-81.

365. Chassevant, M., Richet, C. 1893. Action des sels métalliques sur la fermentation lactique. *Comptes rendus de l'Académie des Sciences*.

366. Héricourt, J., Richet, C. 1893. Tuberculose aviaire et tuberculose humaine chez le singe. *Congres de la Tuberculose*, 281-86.

367. Langlois, J. P., Richet, C. 1893. Une nouvelle fonction du bulbe rachidien; régulation de la température par la respiration. *Travaux du Laboratoire Charles Richet*, Paris: F. Alcan, 431-69.

368. Richet, C. 1893. Etude exp et clinique sur la cocaine. *Travaux du Laboratoire Charles Richet*, Paris: F. Alcan, 529-64.

369. Richet, C. 1893. Le rythme de la respiration. *Physiologie Travaux du Laboratoire* Paris: 55-96.

370. Pachon, V., Richet, C. 1893. De la respiration périodique dans l'intoxication par le chloralose. *Comptes rendus de l'Académie des Sciences*.

371. Richet, C. 1893. Bibliothèque Rétrospective. Marie Théophile Hyacynthe Laennec (1781-1826). De l'auscultation mediate et de l'exploration de la poitrine, Paris: Masson.

372. Richet, C. 1893-1894. La défense de l'organisme. Cours de physiologie de la Faculté de Médecine. Paris: P. Chamerot.

373. Héricourt, J., Richet, C. 1894. Quelques nouveaux exemples de vaccination tuberculose chez le chien. *Comptes rendus Société de Biologie*, Paris (10th ser.) 1:152.

374. Richet, C.: La ralentissement du coeur dans l'asphyxie envisage comme procede de defense. *Bulletin Société de Biologie*, Paris: (10th ser.) 1:243-45.

375. Richet, C. 1894. De la diastase uréopoiétique. *Comptes rendus de la Société de Biologie*, Paris: (10th ser.) 1:525-28.

376. Richet, C. 1894. Le chloralose et ses propriétés hypnotiques. *Review Neurologie* Paris: 2:97-104.

377. Richet, C. 1894. Bibliographia physiologica, Répertoire des travaux de physiologie de l'année 1893-1894; classé d'après la classification décimal . . . ; avec la collaboration de M.M. Athanasiu, J. Carvallo et Dupuy. (5 v). Paris: F. Alcan, Bruxelles: Office Internat. de Bibliog. Zurich, Concilium Bibliog. *Comptes rendus de la Société de Biologie*, Paris: (7th ser.) 4:456-59.

378. Richet, C. 1894. Poids du cerveau, du foie et de la rate, chez l'homme. *Comptes rendus de la Société de Biologie*, Paris: (9th ser.) 6:15-18.

379. Richet, C. 1894. Le frisson musculaire comme procédé thermogène. *Comptes rendus de la Société de Biologie*, Paris (9th ser.) 6:151.

380. Richet, C. 1894. Poids du cerveau, du foie et de la rate des mammifères. *Archives de Physiologie norm. et pathologie*, Paris: (5th ser.) 6:232-45.

381. Richet, C. 1894. La mort du coeur dans l'asphyxie chez le chien. *Archives de Physiologie norm. et Pathologie* Paris: (5th ser.) 6:653-68.

382. Richet, C. 1894. Le chloralose dans l'expérimentation physiologique. *Archives Italian Biologie*, Turin: 21:266-71.

383. Richet, C. 1894. Défense de l'organisme contre les traumatismes. *Revue Scientifique*, 53:259.

384. Richet, C. 1894. Note on the formation of urea in the liver after death. *Med. Press & Cir.* London: (new ser.) 57:667.

385. Richet, C. 1894. De la formation d'urée dans le foie après la mort. *Comptes rendus de l'Académie des Sciences*, Paris: 118:1125-28.

386. Richet, C. 1894. Nagra blad ur Laran om Organesmernas Skyddsmedel. *Revue Finlandaise*, III.

387. Richet, C. 1894-1896. Bibliographia Physiologica, 1893-1894 (1895). Répertoire des travaux de physiologie . . . classés d'après la classification décimale. par. Ch. Richet . . . avec la collaboration de M.M. Athanasiu, J. Carvallo et Dupuy, Paris: F. Alcan. vol. 2.

388. Richet, C. 1894. Exposé des Travaux Scientifiques de M. Charles Richet. Paris: Chamerot et Renouard.

389. Richet, C. 1894. La résistance des canards à l'asphyxie. *Comptes rendus de la Société de Biologie*, Paris: 242-43.

390. Richet, C. 1894. Température maxima observées chez l'homme. *Comptes rendus de la Société de Biologie*, Paris: 416-17.

391. Richet, C. 1895. Dictionnaire de Physiologie, Paris: Anciènne Librairie, Baillière, Vols. 1–10 (1895–1913).

392. Langlois, J. P., Richet, C. 1895. De l'influence de la température sur les convulsions. *Travaux du Laboratoire de Ch. Richet*, Paris: 23–29.

393. Langlois, J. P., Richet, C. 1895. Le frisson comme appareil de régulation therm. *Travaux du Laboratoire de Ch. Richet*, Paris: 23–29.

394. Richet, C. 1895. L'inanition. *Travaux du Laboratoire de Physiologie* Paris: F. Alcan, 301.

395. Lapique, L., Richet, C. 1895. Aliments, Article du Dictionnaire de Physiologie, Paris: 87.

396. Héricourt, J., Richet, C. 1895. Traitement d'un cas de sarcome par la sérotherapie. *Comptes rendus de l'Académie des Sciences*, April.

397. Langlois, J. P., Richet, C. 1895. Radiation calorique après traumatisme de la moelle épinière. *Travaux du Laboratoire Ch. Richet*, Paris: F. Alcan, 415–25.

398. Richet, C. 1896. Jusqu'où, dans l'inanition hystérique, peut aller la privation d'aliments? Des échanges respiratoires dans l'inantion hystérique. *Comptes rendus de la Société de Biologie*, Paris: (10th ser.) 3:945–48.

399. Broca, A., Richet, C. 1896. De la contraction musculaire anaérobie. *Archives Physiologie norm. et Pathologie*, Paris: October, (5th ser.) 8:829–42.

400. Hanriot, M., Richet, C. 1896. Le chloralose. *Archives de Pharmacodynamie*, Paris: 191.

401. Richet, C. 1896–1897. (1850–): Biography Med. Mod. Paris (suppl), 7:125, 1896; also *Revue de l'hypnotique et physiologie* Paris: 11:65–69.

402. Richet, C. 1896. Etudes biologiques sur la douleur. *Revue Scientifique*, Paris: 225–32.

403. Richet, C. 1897. L'oeuvre de Pasteur et la conception moderne de la médecine. *Revue Scientifique*, Paris: 8:417–424; also in *L'Union Médicale*.

404. Richet, C. 1897. La fonction du cerveau. *Revue Scientifique*, Paris: 8:641–49.

405. Richet, C. 1897. The work of Pasteur and the modern conception of medicine. *British Medical Journal*, 56:508–12.

406. Richet, C. 1897. L'oeuvre de Pasteur et la conception moderne de la médecine. *Nature*, 56:508–12.

407. Broca, A., Richet, C. 1897. Période réfractaire dans les centres nerveux. *Comptes rendus de l'Académie des Sciences*, Paris: 124:573–77.

408. Richet, C. 1897. Conspectus methodicus et alphabeticus numerorum. "Systematis decimalis" ad usum bibliographiae physiologicae, confectus autoritate Institutae: Bibliographicae Internationalis Bruxellensis et Societatis Biologicae Parisiensis. Turici: Zurcher & Furrer, 23.

409. Chassevant, A., Richet, C. 1898. Absence du ferment uréopoietique dans le foie des oiseaux. *Comptes rendus de la Société de Biologie*, (10th ser.) 962–63.

410. Richet, C. 1898. Soeur Marthe. Drame lyrique en deux parties, trois actes et cing tableux. Paris: P. Ollendorf, Editeur.

411. Broca, A., Richet, C. 1898. De quelques conditions du travail musculaire chez l'homme. Etude ergométrique. *Archives Physiologie norm. et Pathologie*, (5th ser.) 225–40.

412. Richet, C. 1898. Histoire Universel des Nations.

413. Broca, A., Richet, C, 1899. La vibration nerveuse. *Revue Scientifique*, December.

414. Richet, C., Toulouse. 1899. Influence des sels alkalins de l'alimentation dans le traitement de l'épilepsie. *Comptes rendus de la Société de Biologie*, (10th ser.) December.

415. Richet, C. 1899. Les guérres et la paix, étude sur l'arbitrage international. Paris: Schleicher Frères, 190.

416. Richet, C. 1899. De la resistance des canards à l'asphyxie. Travail du laboratoire de physiologie de la Faculté de Médecine de Paris. *Journal de Physiologie et de Pathologie Générale*, July, 641–50.

417. Richet, C. 1900. Etude historique bibliographique sur l'emploi de la viande crue dans le traitement de la tuberculose. *Semaine Médicale*, 18 July, 1–21.

418. Richet, C. 1900. Douleur. *Dictionnaire de Physiologie*, Paris: Baillière, V. 1, 177.

419. Richet, C. 1900. Défense, fonctions de Dictionnaire de Physiologie. Paris: Baillière, vol. 4, 724.

420. Richet, C. 1900. La thérapéutique expérimentale-thérapéutique metatrophique. *Società Editrice*, Libraria, Milano, 7.

421. Mitchell, C., Richet, C. 1900. De l'accoutumance des ferments aux milieux toxiques. *Comptes rendus de la Société de Biologie*, Paris: 637–39.

422. Langlois, J. P., Richet, C. 1900. De la proportion des chlorures dans les tissues de l'organisme—Influencé de l'alimentation et des autres conditions biologiques. *Journal Physiologie norm. et Pathologie Générale*, September, 743–54.

423. Richet, C. 1900. Foreword to Langlois, J.P. and de Varigny, H.: Nouveaux éléments de physiologie, précédé d'une introduction par Charles Richet, (2d ed) Paris: O. Doin, 912.

424. Richet, C. 1901. Note sur un cas remarquable de précocité musicale. In Janet, P. (ed.) IV Congress Internationel de Psychologie. Paris: F. Alcan, 93–99.

425. Richet, C. 1902. Du poison pruritogène et urticant contenu dans les tentacules des actinies. *Comptes rendus de la Société de Biologie*. Paris: (new ser.) 41:1438–40.

426. Portier, P., Richet, C. 1902. De l'action anaphylactique de certains venins. *Comptes rendus de la Société de Biologie*, Paris: 54:170–72.

427. Portier, P., Richet, C. 1902. Nouveaux faits d'anaphylaxie, ou sensibilisation aux venins par doses réitérées. *Comptes rendus de la Société de Biologie* (1st rep). 13 February.

428. Sully-Prudhomme, M., Richet, C. 1902. Le problème des causes finales. Paris: F. Alcan.

429. Richet, C. 1903–1904. De l'anaphylaxie ou sensibilité croissante des organismes à des doses successives de poison. *Archives di Fisiologie*, Firenze: 1:129–42.

430. Richet, C. 1903. Etude sur un cas de prémonition. *Ann. d. sc. psych.*, Paris: 13:65–71.

431. Richet, C. 1903. Des poisons contenus dans les tentacules des actinies (congestine et thalassine). *Comptes rendus de la Société de Biologie*, Paris: 55:246–48.

432. Richet, C. 1903. L'hypochloruration dans le traitement de l'épilepsie par le bromure de potassium. *Comptes rendus de la Société de Biologie*, Paris: 55:374.

433. Richet, C. 1903. Des ferments protéolytiques et de l'autolyse du foie. *Comptes rendus de la Société de Biologie*, Paris: 55:656–58.

434. Richet, C. 1903. De la thalassine, toxine cristallisée pruritogène. *Comptes rendus de la Société de Biologie*, Paris: 55:707–10.

435. Richet, C. 1903. De la thalassine, considérée comme antitoxine cristallisée. *Comptes rendus de la Société de Biologie*, Paris: 55:1071–73.

436. Richet, C. 1903. Les cultures autogènes. *Comptes rendus de la Société de Biologie,* Paris: 55:1407.
437. Pinard, M.M., Richet, C. 1903. Rapport sur les causes physiologiques de la diminution de la natalité en France. *Ann. de Gynecologie et d'Obstetrique* Paris: 59:15-24.
438. Richet, C. 1903. Foreword to Maxwell, J.: Les phénomènes psychiques; recherches, observations, méthods. Préface de Charles Richet, Paris: F. Alcan, 317.
439. Pinard, M. M., Richet, C. 1903. Rapport sur les causes physiologiques de la diminution de la natalité en France. Melun, Impr. Administrative, 10.
440. Richet, C. 1904. De l'anaphylaxie ou sensibilité croissante des organismes. *Archives di Fisiologie* Firenze: 1:129-42.
441. Richet, C. 1904. La génération spontanée. *Rev. gen. d. sc. pures et appliq.* (2nd ser.) 36:404-11.
442. Richet, C. 1904. Des effets prophylactiques de la thalassine et anaphylactiques de la congestine dans le virus des actinies. *Comptes rendus de la Société de Biologie,* Paris: 56:302.
443. Richet, C. 1904. De l'action des rayons dégagés par le sulfure de calcium phosphrescent sur la fermentation lactique. *Comptes rendus de l'Académie des Sciences,* Paris: 138:588-90.
444. Richet, C. 1904. Etudes sur la fermentation lactique. De l'action soi-disant antiseptique du chloroforme et du benzène. *Comptes rendus de la Société de Biologie,* Paris: 216-19.
445. Richet, C. 1904. Etudes sur la fermentation lactique II. Effets de la fluorescence sur la fermentation lactique. *Comptes rendus de la Société de Biologie,* Paris: 219-21.
446. Richet, C. 1905. Etude sur l'alimentation des chiens tuberculeux. *Revue de Médecine* (25 year) 10 January, 1:1-22.
447. Richet, C. 1905. La personnalité et les changements de la personnalité. *Bulletin de l'Institute Génerale Psychologie,* Paris: 5:113-34.
448. Richet, C. 1905 Faut-il étudier le spiritisme? *Ann. d. sc. psych.,* Paris: 15:1-41.
449. Richet, C. 1905. Notes sur un cas particulier de lucidité. *Ann d. sc. psych.,* Paris: 15:161-66.
450. Richet, C. 1905. Phénomènes métapsychiques d'autrefois. *Ann. d. sc. psych.* Paris: 15:253-77.
451. Richet, C. 1905. La personnalité et les changements de personalité. *Ann. d. sc. psych.,* Paris: 15:253-77.
452. Richet, C. 1905. Xénoglossie; l'écriture automatique en langues étrangères. *Ann. d. sc. psych.,* Paris: 15:317-53; also *Proc. Soc. Psych. Res.,* London: 19:162-266.
453. Richet, C. 1905. De quelques phénomènes dits de matérialisation. *Ann. d. sc. psych.,* Paris: 15:649-71.
454. Richet, C. 1905. Le problème touchant le préjugé des races. *Rev. gen. d. sc. pures et appliq.,* Paris: 16:833-91.
455. Richet, C. 1905. La métapsychique. *Proceedings Sociology Psychology Research,* London: 19:2-49.
456. Richet, C. 1905. Etude sur l'alimentation des chiens tuberculeux. *Revue de Médecine,* Paris: 25:1-22.
457. Richet, C. 1905. Ration alimentaire dans quelques cas de tuberculose humaine. *Revue de Médecine* Paris: 25:97-114.

458. Richet, C. 1905. De l'alimentation dans la tuberculose expérimentale; influence nocive de la viande cuite. *Bulletin Académie de Médecine*, Paris: (3d ser.) 53:593–609; also *Revue de Médecine*, Paris: 25:573–606.

459. Richet, C. 1905. Etudes sur la fermentation lactique; influence de la surface libre sur la marche de la fermentation. *Comptes rendus de la Société de Biologie*, Paris: 57:957–60.

460. Richet, C. 1905. De l'action de la congestine virus des actines sur les lapins et des effets anaphylactiques. *Comptes rendus de la Société de Biologie*, Paris: 58:112–15.

461. Richet, C. 1905. De l'anaphylaxie après injections de congestine, chez le chien. *Comptes rendus de la Société de Biologie*, Paris: 58:16–119.

462. Richet, C. 1905. Anaphylaxie par injections d'apomorphine. *Comptes rendus de la Société de Biologie*, Paris: 58:955–57.

463. Lassablière, P., Lesné, E. and C. Richet. 1905. De l'alimentation par la viande cuite dans la tuberculose expérimentale. *Comptes rendus de la Société de Biologie*, Paris: 58:960–63.

464. Richet, C. 1905. Notzen über thalassin, ein in den Fuhlfaden der Seeneseln befindliches Jucken hervorrufendes Gift. *Arch. f.d. ges physiol.*, Bonn: 108:369–88.

465. Richet, C. 1905. Circé, drame en 2 acts, en vers. (Théatre de Monte Carlo, 2 Avril 1905) Musique de scène de L. Brunel. Paris: J. Gamber, 62.

466. Richet, C. 1905. Conspectus methodicus et alphabeticus numeroroum "systematis decimalis" ad usum bibliographiae physiologicae confectus auctoritate institut: bibliographica internationalis bruxellensis. Ed. nova, ampliata sub auxpiciis. Prof. Caroli Richet ab Dr. H. Jordon. Zurich: Concilium bibliographicum, 73.

467. Richet, C. 1905. Foreword to Joteyko, Mlle J.: Entraînement et fatique au point de vue militaire. Avec préface de Charles Richet, 100, Bruxelles: Misch. & Thron.

468. Richet, C. 1906. Des conditions de la réalimentation après le jeûne. *Zentralb. f.d. ges. physiol. u. path. d. Stoffwechsels*, Berlin: Wien, N.F. 1:161–67.

469. Richet, C. 1906. Infuence de l'émanation du radium sur la fermentation lactique. *Archives Internationale de Physiologie*, Paris: Liége, 3:130–51.

470. Richet, C. 1906. De l'action de doses minuscules de substances sur la fermentation lactique. *Arch. Internationale de Physiology*, Paris: Liége, 3:203–217, 264; also *Comptes rendus de la Société de Biologie*, Paris: 60:981.

471. Lesné, E., Richet, C. 1906. De la ration de lait nécessaire et suffisante chez l'enfant; note sur un procédé d'evaluation. *Arch. de méd. d. enf.*, Paris: 9:449–57.

472. deVesme, C., Richet, C. 1906. Les polémiques du sujet des séances de la Villa Carmen. *Ann. d. sc. psych.*, Paris: 16:129–43.

473. Richet, C. 1906. L'avenir de la psychologie. *Ann. d. sc. psych.* Paris: 16:593–608.

474. Richet, C. 1906. Foreword to: Rouby: Ben Boa et Charles Richet. *Bull. med de l'Algérie*, Alger 17:662–672; 691, 1906; 18:122, 155, 1907; also *Cong. intern. de med.*, Lisbonne: (sect. 7) 15:459–516.

475. Richet, C. 1906. De l'action des métaux a faible dos sur la fermentation lactique. *Comptes rendus de la Société de Biologie*, Paris: 60:455.

476. Richet, C. 1906. Expériences sur les alternances de jeûne et d'alimentation chez les lapins. *Comptes rendus de la Société de Biologie*, Paris: 61:546–48.

477. Richet, C. 1906. De l'action toxique de la subértine (extrait aqueux de Subérites domuncula). *Comptes rendus de la Société de Biologie*, Paris: 61:589–600.

478. Richet, C. 1906. De la variabilité de la dose toxique de suberitine. *Comptes rendus de la Société de Biologie*, Paris: 61:686–88.
479. Richet, C. 1906. Effets reconstituants de la viande crue après le jeûne. *Comptes rendus de l'Académie des Sciences*, Paris: 142:522–24.
480. Richet, C. 1906. Peace and War. Translated from the French by Marion Edwards. London: J.M. Dent & Co.
481. Richet, C. 1906. Les phénomènes dits de matérialisation de la Villa Carmen avec documents nouveaux et discussion. *Ann. des Sciences Psychiques*, Paris.
482. Richet, C. 1906. Sur une combinaison de l'acide lactique avec la caséine dans la fermentation lactique. *Comptes rendus de la Société de Biologie*, Paris: 650–651.
483. Richet, C. 1907. Les bases psychologiques de la morale. *Bulletin de l'Institute Génerale Psychologie*, Paris: 7:3–33.
484. Richet, C. 1907. De l'anaphylaxie dans l'intoxication par la cocaine. *Archives Internationale de Pharmacologie et Therapie*, Paris: 18:2–14.
485. Richet, C. 1907. De l'anaphylaxie en générale et de l'anaphylaxie par la mytilocongestine en particulier. *Annals de l'Institute Pasteur*, Paris: 21:497–524.
486. Richet, C. 1907. Anaphylaxie par la mytilocongestine. *Comptes rendus de la Société de Biologie*, Paris: 62:358–60.
487. Richet, C. 1907. Mesure de l'anaphylaxie par la dose émétisante. *Comptes rendus de la Société de Biologie*, Paris: 62:643–45.
488. Richet, C. 1907. Le passé de la guerre et l'avenir de la Paix. Paris: Ollendorf.
489. Richet, C. 1908. An enquiry into premonitions. *Ann. Psych. Sc.*, London: 7:24–26.
490. Richet, C. 1908. Ueber die Wirkung schwacher Dosen auf physiologische Vörgange und auf die Garungen im besorderen. *Biochem. ztscher*, Berlin: 11:273–80.
491. Richet, C. 1908. De l'anaphylaxie. *Presse Médecine*. Paris: 16:185–87.
492. Richet, C. 1908. De l'anaphylaxie et des toxogénines. *Annals de l'Institute Pasteur*, Paris: 22:465–95.
493. Richet, C. 1908. La médecine, les médecins et les Facultés de Médecine. *Revue des Deux Mondes*, Paris: 5 per., 45:541–675, 1 June.
494. Richet, C. 1908. De la substance anaphylactisante ou toxogénine. *Comptes rendus de la Société de Biologie*, Paris: 64:846–48.
495. Richet, C. 1908. De la variation de la température organique des chiens selon le pelage. *Comptes rendus de la Société de Biologie*, Paris: 64:880.
496. Richet, C. 1908. The pros and cons of vivisection, by Dr. Charles Richet . . . with a preface by W.D. Halliburton, London: Duckworth & Co., 136.
497. Richet, C. 1908. Note sur l'anaphylaxie. Des proprietes differentes dissociables par la chaleur d'une substance toxique. *Comptes rendus de la Société de Biologie*, Paris.
498. Richet, C. 1909. Etudes sur la crépitine (toxine de Hura crepitans). *Annals de l'Institute Pasteur*, Paris: 23:745–800.
499. Richet, C. 1909. Du poison contenu dans la sève du Hura crepitans (ou assaku). *Comptes rendus de la Société de Biologie*, Paris: 66:763.
500. Richet, C. 1909. L'anaphylaxie crée d'un poison nouveau chez l'animal sensibilisé. *Comptes rendus de la Société de Biologie*, Paris: 66:810.
501. Richet, C. 1909. De la réaction anaphylactique in vitro. *Comptes rendus de la Société de Biologie*, Paris: 66:1005–07.
502. Lassablière, P., Richet, C. 1909. Leucocytose prolongée apres intoxication. *Comptes rendus de la Société de Biologie*, Paris: 67:782.

503. Lassablière, P. and C. Richet. 1909. Action du sulfure de calcium phosphorescent sur le fermentation lactique. *Travaux du Laboratoire*, de Ch. Richet, Paris: F. Alcan, 19-73.

504. Richet, C. 1909. Die Vergangenheit des Krieges und die zukunft des Friedens. Autorisierte Übersetzung von Bertha V. Suttner. Wien: Osterreichische Friedensgesellschaft, 255.

505. Richet, C. 1909. Observations relatives au vol des oiseaux, 303-21.

506. Richet, C. 1909. Le passé de la guerre et l'avenir de la paix. Paris.

507. Richet, C. 1909 Rôle du Système Nerveux dans les Phénomènes de l'anaphylaxie Aigué. *Presse Médecine* Mercredi 7 Avril.

508. Nogues, P., Richet, C. 1910. Expériences sur le vol des pigeons à ailes rognés. *Travaux Association de l'Institute Marey*, Paris: 2:217-24.

509. Richet, C. 1910. L'humorisme ancien et moderne. *Presse Médecine*, Paris: 18:729-33; also translated *British Medical Journal*, London: 2:921-26.

510. Richet, C. 1910. L'anaphylaxie. *J. Méd. Franc.*, Paris: 4:379-83.

511. Richet, C. 1910. Obituary of Angelo Mosso (1846-1910). Necrology. *Rev. gen. d. sc. pures et appliq.*, Paris: 21:1001.

512. Richet, C. 1910. Nouvelles expériences sur la crépitine et l'actino-congestine (anaphylaxie et immunité). *Annals de l'Institute Pasteur*, Paris: 24:609-52.

513. Richet, C. 1910. Die Humorallehre in der alten und modernen Physiologie. *Wiener Med. Woch.*, 60:2353-66.

514. Richet, C. 1910. Notes statistiques sur la progression des memoires et travaux de physiologie. *Comptes rendus de la Société de Biologie*, Paris: 68:401.

515. Richet, C. 1910. Protoxines et transformations des protoxines. *Comptes rendus de la Société de Biologie*, Paris: 68:500-2.

516. Richet, C. 1910. Accroissement générale de la sensibilité aux poisons chez les animaux anaphylactisés. *Comptes rendus de la Société de Biologie*, Paris: 68:820.

517. Richet, C. 1910. De la séroanaphylaxie homogénique. *Comptes rendus de la Société de Biologie*, Paris: 69:2-4.

518. Richet, C. 1910. De la loi biologique qui gouverne la toxicité des corps simples. *Comptes rendus de la Société de Biologie*, Paris: 69:433-35.

519. Richet, C. 1910. L'humorisme ancien et l'humorisme moderne discours prononcé au congrès de physiol. de Vienne, Paris: Masson, 25 September, 42.

520. Richet. C. 1911. De l'anaphylaxie alimentaire par la crépitine. *Annals de l'Institute Pasteur*, Paris: 25:580-92.

521. Richet, C. 1911. L'anaphylaxie et la finalité. *Revue de Médecine*. Paris: 31:719-22.

522. Richet, C. 1911. De l'anaphylaxie alimentaire. *Comptes rendus de la Société de Biologie*, Paris: 70:44-48.

523. Richet, C. 1911. Immunité antianaphylaxie et leucocytose, après ingestion. *Comptes rendus de la Société de Biologie*, Paris: 70:252.

524. Lassablière, P., Richet, C. 1911. De la leucocytose dans la zomothérapie (alimentation avec le jus de viande crue). *Comptes rendus de la Société de Biologie*, Paris: 70:945-47

525. Richet, C. 1911. Influence de la rate sur la nutrition. *Comptes rendus de la Société de Biologie*, Paris: 71:635-37.

526. Richet, C. 1911. L'anaphylaxie. F. Alcan, Paris: 286.

527. Lassablière, P., Richet, C. 1911. Leucocytes digestive après ingestion de viande (cuite ou crue). *Comptes rendus de la Société de Biologie*, LXX:637, 29 April.

528. Lassablière, P., Richet, C. 1912. La leucocytose produits par l'injection intrapéritonéale d'albumine out de peptone est indépendante de la dose. *Comptes rendus de la Société de Biologie*, Paris: 72:944.

529. Lassabliére, P., Richet, C. 1912. Persistance de la leucocytose après une injection de peptone. *Comptes rendus de la Société de Biologie*, Paris: 72:945.

530. Richet, C. 1912. De la durée prolongée dans l'anaphylaxie alimentaire. *Comptes rendus de la Société de Biologie*, Paris: 72:947.

531. Lassablière, P., Richet, C. 1912. De la leucocytose provoqué par les injections péritonéales. *Comptes rendus de la Société de Biologie*, Paris: 73:520.

532. Lassablière, P., Richet, C. 1912. Immunité élémentaire après injections péritonéales. *Comptes rendus de la Société de Biologie*, Paris: 73:542-44.

533. Richet, C. 1912. Abrégé d'histoire générale. Paris: Hachette.

534. Richet, C. 1912. Mélanges Biologiques (Jubilée) de C. Richet) Paris: Imprimerie de la Cour D'Appel.

535. Richet, C. 1912. Foreword to Le Play. *Technique opératoire phys. tube digestif.* Paris.

536. Richet, C. 1913. De la délimitation de l'anaphylaxie. *J. méd. Franc.* Paris: 7:14-18.

537. Richet, C. 1913. La réaction leucocytaire; digestion, intoxication; immunité. *Presse Médecine.* Paris: 21:537-40.

538. Lassablière, P., Richet, C. 1913. De l'immunité leucocytaire. *Comptes rendus de la Société de Biologie*, Paris: 74:746-50.

539. Laugier, H., Richet, C. 1913. Les variations du temps de réaction (équation personnelle) au cours du travail professionel. *Comptes rendus de la Société de Biologie*, Paris: 74:816-19.

540. Lassablière, P., Richet, C. 1913. De l'immunité (leucocytaire) générale. *Comptes rendus de la Société de Biologie*, Paris: 74:1167.

541. Richet, C. 1913. Une race de ferment lactique arsénicophile (accoutumée aux doses fortes d'arsenic). *Comptes rendus de la Société de Biologie*, Paris: 74:1252-54.

542. Richet, C. 1913. Des effets de l'ablation de la rate sur la nutrition chez les chiens. *Journal de Physiologie et de Pathologie Génerale*, 1, XIV:689-703, July; also deuxièm Mémoire 1, XV: May, 1913.

543. Richet, C. 1913. Anaphylaxis (translated by Murray Bligh). Liverpool: University Presses.

544. Richet, C. 1913. Dictionnaire de Physiologie, Anciènne Librairie, Germer Baillière, vol. 9, Paris: 1895-1913.

545. Richet, C. 1913. Theories of immunity and anaphylaxis. L'anaphylaxie alimentaire. *Transactions International Congress Medicine London* (sec IV, Bacteriol. & Immun), 13-128.

546. Lassablière, P., Richet, C. 1914. Influence du froid sur la leucocytose. *Comptes rendus de la Société de Biologie*, Paris: 76:39.

547. Richet, C. 1914. Biography. *Gazette Médecine de Paris*, (annexe) 85:iii.

548. Richet, C. 1914. Un nouveau type d'anaphylaxie; l'anaphylaxie indirecte: leucocytose et chloroforme. *Comptes rendus de l'Académie des Sciences*, Paris: 158:304-8.

549. Richet, C. 1914. De la non accoutumance héréditaire des microorganismes (ferment lactique) aux milieux peu nutritifs. *Comptes rendus de l'Académie des Sciences*, Paris: 158:1749-53.

550. Richet, C. 1914. Foreword to Maxwell, J.: Les Phénomènes Psychiques.

551. Richet, C. 1915. Adaptation des microbes (ferment lactique au milieu). *Annals de l'Institute Pasteur*, Paris: 29:22–54.

552. Richet, C. 1915. Notice (Obituary) sur Justus Lucas-Championnière (1842–1913), *J. de m., et chir. prat.*, Paris: 86:481–453 also in *Revue Scientifique*, Paris: 1:353–58.

553. Richet, C. 1915. De l'action stimulante des sels de magnésium sur la fermentation lactique. *Comptes rendus d l'Académie des Sciences*, Paris: 161:264.

554. Richet, C. 1916. La science Française. Descartes, Lavoisier, Pasteur. Revue Scientifique, Paris: 1:357–62.

555. Richet, C. 1916. Le courage. *Revue Scientifique*, Paris: 2:385–91.

556. Richet, C. 1916. Etude clinique et bactériologique des entérites chloroformes observées au Cap Helles. *Paris Médecine*, 18:361–67.

557. Richet, C. 1916. Les évenements psychiques de la guerre. Un appel de M. Charles Richet aux soldats; avez-vous des pressentiments? *Ann. d. sc. Psych.*, Paris: 26:185–92.

558. Richet, C. 1916. De la variation mensuelle de la natalité. *Comptes rendus de l'Académie des Sciences*, Paris: 163:141–49.

559. Richet, C. 1916. Des conditions qui influent sur l'écart mensuel moyen de la natalité. *Comptes rendus de l'Académie des Sciences*, Paris: 163:161–66.

560. Richet, C. 1916. De l'emploi alternant des antiseptiques. *Comptes rendus de l'Académie des Sciences*, Paris: 163:589.

561. Richet, C. 1916. Les Coupables. Flammarion, 271.

562. Richet, C. 1917. Obituary: A. Dastre (1843–1917) Biography. *Journal de Physiologie et de Pathologie génenerale*, Paris: 17: p.v.

563. Gley, E., Tessier, P., Richet, C. 1917. Obituary Jules Courmont (1865–1917) Portrait. *Journal de Physiologie et Pathologie Générale*, Paris: 17:1–11.

564. Richet, C. 1917. La fermentation lactique et les sels de thallium; étude sur l'héredité. *Annals de l'Institute Pasteur*, Paris: 31:51–59.

565. Richet, C. 1917. Dépopulation of France. *Annals de Gynecologie et d'Obstetrique*, 72:577 (July-August); also *Bulletin Académie de Médecine*, Paris: (3d ser.) 77:604–634; (Discussion) 691, 716, 756, 781.

566. Richet, C. 1917. Declining birth rate. *Bulletin Académie de Médecine*, Paris: 78:396 (16 October) 78:441 (23 October).

567. Richet, C. 1917. Classification of antiseptics. *Bulletin Académie de Médecine*, Paris: 78:425 (16 October).

568. Cardot, H., LeRolland, P., Richet, C. 1917. Des antiseptiques réguliers et irréguliers. *Comptes rendus de l'Académie des Sciences*, Paris: 164:669–74.

569. Cardot, H., Richet, C. 1917. D'un nouveau procédé de dosage des matières reductrices de l'urine. *Comptes rendus de l'Académie des Sciences*, Paris: 165:258–62.

570. Cardot, H., Richet, C. 1917. Des antiseptiques réguliers et irréguliers. *Comptes rendus de l'Académie des Sciences*, Paris: 165:491–96; also *Bulletin Académie de Médecine* Paris: (3d ser.) 78:425–27.

571. Richet, C., Brodin, P., Saint-Girons, F. 1918. Influence des injections intraveineuses de liquides isotoniques sur la dilution du sang et sur le nombre des hematies qui peuvent etre perdus dans les hémorragies. *Comptes rendus d l'Académie des Sciences*, Paris: 1:166, 664, 669, 29 April.

572. Richet, C. 1918. Intravenous injections after hemorrhage. *Presse Médecine*, (14 November) 26:581.

573. Richet, C., Brodin, P., Saint-Girons, F. 1918. Effets des injections intraveineuses des divers serums artificiels chez les animaux hémorragies. *Presse Médecine*, Paris: 26:581-82.

574. Richet, C. 1918. Des variations individuelles de l'azote urinaire. *Comptes rendus de la Société de Biologie*. Paris: 81:133-35.

575. Richet, C. 1918. Des variations individuelles de l'azote urinaire. *Comptes rendus de la Société de Biologie*. Paris: 81:255.

576. Brodin, P., Saint-Girons, F., Richet, C. 1918. Densité hématies, leucocytes, et quantité de sang chez 47 chiens à l'état normal. *Comptes rendus de la Société de Biologie*, Paris: 81:681-84.

577. Cardot, H., Richet, C. 1918. De l'action des mélanges de quelques sels sur la fermentation lactique. *Comptes rendus de la Société de Biologie*, Paris: 81:751-55.

578. Noizet, G., Richet, C. 1918. Influence de la compression des membres inférieurs et de l'abdomen sur la pression artérielle dans l'aorte superieure. *Comptes rendus de la Société de Biologie*, Paris: 81:804-6.

579. Richet, C., Brodin, P., Saint-Girons, F. 1918. De la densité du sang après les grandes hémorragies. *Comptes rendus de l'Académie des Sciences*, Paris: 166:587-93.

580. Richet, C., Flament, L. 1918. De quelques troubles de la sécrétion urinaire après les grands traumatismes. *Comptes rendus de l'Académie des Sciences*, Paris: 166:718-22.

581. Richet, C., Brodin, P., and Saint-Girons, F. 1918. De quelques modifications au traitement de la tuberculose pulmonaire par les inhalations antiseptiques. *Comptes rendus de l'Académie des Sciences*, Paris: 166:92-94.

582. Richet, C. 1918. A propos de la plasmothérapie (dans le traitement de la grippe). *Comptes rendus de l'Académie des Sciences*, Paris: 167-766.

583. Richet, C. 1918. L'anesthésie générale par le chloralose dans le cas de choc traumatique et d'hémorragie. *Comptes rendus de l'Académie des Sciences*, Paris: 1026-34.

584. Richet, C., Brodin, P., Saint-Girons, F. 1918. Nouvelles observations sur les effets des transfusions salines intraveineuses après hémorragies graves. *Comptes rendus de l'Académie des Sciences*, Paris: 167:112-15.

585. Richet, C., Brodin, P., Saint-Girons, F. 1918. Effets des injections intraveineuses isotoniques dans les hémorragies. *Comptes rendus de l'Académie des Sciences*, Paris: 167:55-59.

586. Brodin, P., Richet, C. 1918. Ohmhémomètre pour mesurer la résistivité électrique du sang; application à la clinique. *Comptes rendus de l'Académie des Sciences*, Paris: 167:413-18.

587. Richet, C., Brodin, P., Saint-Girons, F. 1918. Survie temporaire et survie définitive après les hémorragies graves. *Comptes rendus de l'Académie des Sciences*, Paris: 167:574-79.

588. Richet, C. 1918. Les coupables, Paris: Flammarion, 2d ed.

589. Richet, C. 1918. War Nursing. What Every Woman Should Know. Translated by Helen De Vere Beauclerk, London: Wm. Heinemann.

590. Richet, C. 1918. L'anesthésie dans les blessures de guerre Fermin-Didot et cie, Paris: MDCCCCXVIII (1918). Presented at the Annual Public Meeting of the 5 Academies, 25 October.
591. Barbier, A., Richet, C. 1919. Contributions à l étude bactériologique des infections aérobies dans les complications bronchiques ou pulmonaires de la grippe. Importance des associations microbiénnes. *Annals de Médecine*, Paris: 6:37-49.
592. Brodin, P., Richet, C., Saint-Girons, F. 1919. Nombres relatifs et absolus des leucocytes à l'état normal et dans les hémorragies chez le chien. *Journal de Physiologie et Pathologie Génerale*, Paris: 18:27-32.
593. Brodin, P., Richet, C., Saint-Girons, F. 1919. De la quantité de sang (masse de sang) mesurée par le nombre des hématies. *Journal de Physiologie et de Pathologie Generale*, Paris: 18:8-26.
594. Richet, C. 1919. Les maîtres de la physiologie. I. Descartes, Lavoisier, *Presse Médecine*, Paris: 27:257.
595. Richet, C. 1919. Les maîtres de la physiologie. II. Claude Bernard, Pasteur, *Presse Médecine*, Paris: 27:297-99.
596. Richet, C. 1919. Lucidité. *Ann. d. sc. psych.*, Paris: 29:51-53.
597. Cardot, H., Richet, C. 1919. Hérédité accoutumance et variabilité dans la fermentation lactique. *Annals de l'Institute Pasteur*, Paris: 33:575-615.
598. Richet, C. 1919. L'anesthésie dans les blessures de la guèrre. *Revue Scientifique*. Paris: 57:161-65.
599. Richet, C. 1919. Obituary: François Henri Hallopeau (1842-1919). *Comptes rendus de la Société de Biologie*, Paris: 82:257.
600. Richet, C. 1919. De la prévision de la température dans les maladies fébriles. *Comptes rendus de la Société de Biologie*, Paris: 82:365.
601. Richet, C. 1919. L'alimentation avec les aliments stérilisés. Remarque à propos de la note de M. Wollman. *Comptes rendus de la Société de Biologie*, Paris: 82:601.
602. Richet, C. 1919. Obituary: Luigi Luciani (1842-1919). *Comptes rendus de la Société de Biologie*, Paris: 82:1214.
603. Brodin, P., Richet, C., Saint-Girons, F. 1919. Des phénomenes hématiques dans l'anaphylaxie et l'antianaphylaxie (crise hémo-anaphylactique). *Comptes rendus de l'Académie des Sciences*, Paris: 168:369-76.
604. Noizet, G., Richet, C. 1919. D'un vêtement insubersible et protecteur contre le froid. *Comptes rendus de l'Académie des Sciences*, Paris: 168:534-36.
605. Richet, C. 1919. Injections de gomme ou de plasma après hémorragie. *Comptes rendus de l'Académie des Sciences*, Paris: 169:1072-74.
606. Brodin, P., Richet, C., Saint-Girons, F. 1919. De l'action immunisante du chlorure de sodium contre l'injection anaphylactique déchainante (thérapeutique metatrophique). *Comptes rendus de l'Académie des Sciences*, Paris: 169:9-16.
607. Richet, C. 1919. L'homme stupide. Paris: E. Flammarion. 220.
608. Richet, C. 1919. La sélection humaine. Paris: F. Alcan, 262.
609. Richet, C. 1919. Abrégé d'histoire générale. Essai sur le passé de l'homme et des sociétés humaines. Paris: Hachette, 600.
610. Richet, C. 1920. Experimental research on antiseptics. *Médecine*, Paris: 1:719 (September).
611. Richet, C. 1920. Les prémonitions, no. 1, 18-26, no. 2, 74-80, *Revue Scientifique*, Paris.

612. Richet, C., Brodin, P., Saint-Girons, F. 1920. Une nouvelle méthode d'antianaphylaxie (méthode metatrophique). *Review de Médecine*, Paris: 37:7-15.
613. Cardot, H., Richet, C. 1920. De l'échauffement du foie post mortem par l'électrisation. *Comptes rendus de la Société de Biologie*, Paris: 83:142.
614. Cardot, H., Richet, C. 1920. La transmission héréditaire des caractères acquis et l'accoutumance des microbes. *Comptes rendus de l'Académie des Sciences*, Paris: 171:1353-58.
615. Richet, C. 1920. Ce que toute femme doit savoir, Leçons de physiologie élémentaire, Paris: F. Alcan.
616. Richet, C. 1920. Travaux de laboratoire de physiologie. Paris: F. Alcan.
617. Richet, C. 1921. Anaphylaxie, its rôle and its treatment; a study of poisons that made the victim more sensitive to a second degree. *Scientific American*, New York: 4:221-24.
618. Richet, C., Bachrach, E. 1921. Accoutumance et sélection du ferment lactique dans les milieux toxiques. *Journal de Physiologie et de Pathologie Génerale*, Paris: 19:466-79.
619. Richet, C. 1921. Anaphylaxie et finalité. *Scientia*, Bologna (2d ser.) 29:275-80.
620. Richet, C., Bachrach, E. and H. Cardot. 1921. Les phénomènes d'anaphylaxie chez les microbes. *Comptes rendus de l'Académie des Sciences*, Paris: 172:512-14.
621. Richet, C., Bachrach, E., Cardot, H. 1921. Les alternances entre l'accoutumance et l'anaphylaxie (Etude sur le ferment lactique). *Comptes rendus de l'Académie des Sciences*, Paris: 172:1554-57.
622. Richet, C. 1921. L'unité psychologique du temps. *Comptes rendus de l'Académie des Sciences*, Paris: 173:1313-27.
623. Richet, C. 1921. Les ténébres de l'heure. Fragments de poésie. Paris: F. Alcan.
624. Richet, C., Sr. and C. Richet, Jr. 1921. Traité de physiologie médico-chirurgicale. 2 v. 1452 paged consec., Paris: F. Alcan.
625. Richet, C. 1922. Birth rate in France. *Médecine*, 3:810-13, August.
626. Richet, C. 1922. Des moyennes en physiologie. *Arch. nederl. de physiol.*, La Haye 7:31-38.
627. Richet, C. 1922. La Gloire de Pasteur. Supplément to *La Vie Médicale*, 104-106; also *Paris Médecine* (annexe) 46:422-45; also (poem) *Semana Médecine*. 2:1326-28, 28 December.
628. Richet, C. 1922. Le centenaire de Pasteur. *Comptes rendus de la Société de Biologie*, Paris: 87:1309-13.
629. Richet, C., Bachrach, E. and H. Cardot. 1922. Accoutumance du ferment lactique aux poisons (Spécificité, simultanéité et alternance. *Comptes rendus de l'Académie des Sciences*, Paris: 174:345-51.
630. Richet, C., Bachrach, E. and H. Cardot. 1922. Etudes sur la fermentation lactique. Le souvenir chez les microbes. *Comptes rendus de l'Académie des Sciences*, Paris: 174:842-45.
631. Richet, C., LeBer, Mme. A.G. 1922. Etudes sur la fermentation lactique. Action a très faibles doses de substance en apparence inoffensives. *Comptes rendus de l'Académie des Sciences*, Paris: 175:1021-24.
632. Richet, C. 1922. L'hypothèse spirite; Réponse à Sir Oliver Lodge. *Revue Métapsychique*, no. 3, 153-57.

633. Richet, C. 1922. Expériences décisives de cryptesthésie (lucidité). *Revue Métapsychique*, no. 3, 158–67.
634. Richet, C. 1922. A propos des ectoplasmes. *Revue Métapsychique*, no. 5, 281–83.
635. Richet, C. 1922. L'hypothèse de l'hyperesthésie tactile dans les expériences d'Ossowiecki. *Revue Métapsychique*, no. 5, 299–300.
636. Richet, C. 1922. (with R. Santoliquido and A. de Gramont): Le campagne d'injures et de mensonges: Declaration du comité. *Revue Métapsychique*, no. 6. 353.
637. Richet, C. 1922. De la théorie spirite: Réponse a M. Bozzano, *Revue Métapsychique*, no. 6, 366–71.
638. Richet, C. 1922. Un dernier mot sur la cryptesthésie, lucidité: Réponse à M. Bozzano. *Revue Métapsychique*, no. 6, 382–84.
639. Richet, C. 1922. Traité de métapsychique. Paris: F. Alcan.
640. Richet, C. 1923. Extrasensorial channels of knowledge and experimental method. *Lancet*, 2:493–497 (8 September).
641. Richet, C. 1923. Métapsychique. *Presse Médecine*, 31:937–40 (10 November).
642. Richet, C. 1923. Work of Pasteur. *Review de Médecine*, 40:257–272 (May); 40:33–353 (June); 40:405–31 (July).
643. Richet, C. 1923. La rate, organe utile, non nécessaire. *Comptes rendus de l'Académie des Sciences*, Paris: 176:1026–31.
644. Garrelon, L., Santenoise, D., Richet, C. 1923. Le réflexe laryngo-cardiaque. *Comptes rendus de l'Académie des Sciences*, Paris: 176:347–50.
645. Richet, C. 1923. Role de la rate dans la nutrition. *Comptes rendus de l'Académie des Sciences*, Paris: 176:1581–83.
646. Richet, C. 1923. Influence de l'ablation de la rate dans les cas d'alimentation défectueuse. *Comptes rendus de l'Académie des Sciences*, 177:441–44.
647. Richet, C. 1923. An address on extra sensorial channels of knowledge and the experimental method. *Lancet*, 493:497.
648. Richet, C. 1923. L'oeuvre de Pasteur. Paris: F. Alcan, 118.
649. Richet, C. 1923. Le Savant, par le Prof. Charles Richet . . . Paris: Hachette, 128.
650. Richet, C. 1923. Chez Victor Hugo. *Revue Métapsychique*, no. 3, 137–52.
651. Richet, C. 1923. *Dictionnaire de Physiologie*, Paris: F. Alcan, Vol. 9–10, 287.
652. Richet, C. 1923. Les Médecins sociologiques et hommes d'état par Prisca (Pètre) Paris: F. Alcan, IV–24; 19 cm, Bibliogr. 205–22.
653. Richet, C. 1923. Thirty years of psychical research; being a treatise on metapsychics. transl. from the French by Stanley De Brath, New York: Macmillan & Co., 646.
654. Richet, C. 1923. Traité de Métapsychique. Paris: F. Alcan, 748–85.
655. Richet, C. 1923. Traité de physiologie médico-chirurgicale. Paris: F. Alcan (Unter Mitarbeit von Charles Richet fils).
656. Richet, C. 1923. Gundriss der Parapsychologie und Parapsychophysik. Mit einem Geleitwort von Dr. Albert Freiherrn von Schrenk-Notzing. Ins. Deutsch ubertragen von Rudolf Lamber, 491, Stuttgart, Berlin, Leipzig.
657. Richet, C. 1924. La défense de la métapsychique; Réponse au Docteur Achille Delmas. *Revue Métapsychique*, Paris: No. 1 1:5–16.
658. Richet, C. 1924. Lécriture "presque" automatique. *Revue Métapsychique*, Paris: No. 2, 2:135–37.
659. Richet, C. 1924. Normal Life. *Médecine* 5:912–16, (September).
660. Cardot, H., Richet, C. 1924. Method for estimating lactic fermentation. *Annals de l'Institute Pasteur*, 38:842–47 (September).

661. Richet, C. 1924. Obituary. Emile Wertheimer (1852-1924). *Comptes rendus de la Société de Biologie*, Paris: 91:1060.
662. Richet, C. 1924. Le jus de viande cru, pur, sec, et total dans le traitement de la tuberculose humaine et la réconstruction des muscles. *Comptes rendus de l'Académie des Sciences*, Paris: 178:1660-66.
663. Richet, C. 1924. Initiation à l'histoire de la France et de la civilisation Française. Paris: Hachette, 187.
664. Richet, C. 1924. La Nouvelle Zomothérapie, thérapeutique, expérimentale et clinique. par Charles Richet, Paris: Masson, 223.
665. Richet, C. 1925. Obituary: Jean Camus (1872-1924). Presse méd., Paris: 33, 28.
666. Richet, C. 1925. Métapsychics. *Presse Médecine*, 33:857-62 (27 June).
667. Richet, C. 1925. L'oeuvre du lab de Physiol. de la Faculté de Médecine, 1881-1925, *Presse Médecine*, 33:1009-12, 29 July.
668. Richet, C. 1925. Radiographies pour le diagnostic de la nature du travail humain exécuté sur les dents en ethnographie. *Comptes rendus de l'Académie des Sciences*, Paris: 181:1091.
669. Richet, C. 1925. Effets des sels de zirconium, de titane et de maganèse sur la nutrition. *Comptes rendus de l'Académie des Sciences*, Paris: 181:1105.
670. Richet, C. 1925. La danse automatique. *Revue Métapsychique*, No. 1, 37-38.
671. Richet, C. 1925. Camille Flammarion. *Revue Métapsychique*, no. 3, 129-31.
672. Richet, C. 1925. Mes deux derniéres Leçons. Paris: Masson.
673. Richet, C. 1925. Idiot man or the follies of mankind (translated by Norah Forsythe and Lloyd Harvey). London: Werner Laure.
674. Richet, C. 1925. Compendio de historia universal, ensayo sobre el pasado del hombre y de las sociedades humanas. Prefactio de la edicion espanola de Angel Puliod. Barcelona: Casa editorial Araluce.
675. Richet, C. 1926. Un problème de biologie générale: à propos de nouvelles expèriences de cryptesthésie. *Revue Métapsychique*, Paris: 1:26-27.
676. Richet, C. 1926. Une critique inopérante: M. Albert Moll et la cryptesthésie de Kahn, *Revue Métapsychique*, Paris: 3:215-18.
677. Richet, C. 1926. Histoire de la circulation de Michel Servet à William Harvey. Esculape, Paris: (new ser.) 16:49-55.
678. Lassablière, P., Richet, C. 1926. Effets protecteurs du chloralose sur l'anesthésie chloroformique. *Comptes rendus de l'Académie des Sciences*, Paris: 183:175.
679. Richet, C. 1926. De l'accoutumance des poissons marins aux eaux sursaturées. *Comptes rendus de l'Académie des Sciences*, Paris: 183:627-29.
680. Richet, C. 1926. The new zomotherapy. Paris; Richon et Flourdeau.
681. Richet, C. 1926. Au Docteur Auguste Pettit. Paris: *Editions Médicales*, Paris: 14.
682. Richet, C. 1926. Aux jeunes gens des écoles de tous les pays. Histoire universelle des civilisations, par M. Charles Richet . . . la Flèche: Depot des publications de la concilation, 86.
683. Lassablière, P., Richet, C. 1926. Effets protecteurs des injections salines préalables sur l'anesthésie chloroformique. *Comptes rendus de l'Académie des Sciences*, Paris: 182.
684. Richet, C. 1927. Une citation de la Bruyère. *Revue Métapsychique*, 2:126.
685. Richet, C. 1927. Physiologie Comparée - Des conditions de la mort par le tétanose électrique chez les poissons. *Comptes rendus de l'Académie des Sciences*, 184:1100-03.

686. Richet, C. 1927. L'homme Impuissant. Arch. D'Imprimerie Le 15 Févier, *Editions Montaigne*, 197.

687. Richet, C. 1927. L'intelligence et l'homme; études de psychologie et de physiologie. Paris: F. Alcan.

688. Richet, C. 1927. The natural history of a savant (translated by Sir Oliver Lodge) London: Dent.

689. Richet, C. 1928. Review of Die Grundprobleme der Astrologie, by K.T. Bayer, *Revue Métapsychique*, 1:71–72.

690. Richet, C. 1928. Y a-t-il une fatalité aux choses? *Revue Métapsychique*, 3:223.

691. Richet, C. 1928. Monition d'un fait vraisemblable. *Revue Métapsychique*, 3:224.

692. Richet, C. 1928. Les prévisions de l'avenior aujourd'hui à il y mille ans. *Revue Métapsychique*, 4:255–62.

693. Richet, C. 1928. A propos du "sixième sens: Réponse à M. le Dr. Osty. *Revue Métapsychique*, 5:398–99.

694. Richet, C., Menetrier, P. 1928. Claude Bernard. *Progres Médecine*, 43:209–40 (11 February).

695. Richet, C. 1928. Pour les petits, Fables, illustrées par Marius Chambon, Paris: J. Peyronnet, 106.

696. Richet, C. 1928. Pour les grands et les petits. Fables. Paris: O. Doin: 176.

697. Richet, C. 1928. Notre sixieme sens. Paris: Montaigne, 253.

698. Richet, C. 1929. A de Schrenk-Notzing. *Revue Métapsychique*, 2:73–76.

699. Richet, C. 1929. Review of *Quand la Navire.* by Jules Romains, *Revue Métapsychique,* 5:456–459.

700. Richet, C., (Mme.) L. Braumann. 1929. Action accélérante des sels de lanthane à dose très faible sur la fermentation. *Comptes rendus de l'Académie des Sciences,* Paris: 188:1198 (6 May).

701. Richet, C. 1929. Our Sixth Sense; transl; by F. Rothwell. Rider, 227.

702. Richet, c. 1929. Apologie de la biologie. Paris: O. Doin, 84.

703. Richet, C. 1929. The Impotence of Man. Translated by Lloyd Harvey. Boston: Stratford.

704. Richet, C. 1930. Le métapsychique oriental et son meant. *Revue Métapsychique*, 1:1–4.

705. Richet, C. 1930. Deux monitions? *Revue Métapsychique* 1:71–72.

706. Richet, C. 1930. Rève monitoire par un enfant. *Revue Métapsychique*, 3:262–63.

707. Richet, C. 1930. A propos a Thérèsa Neumann: Les jeûnes prolongés. *Revue Métapsychique*, 3:385–95.

708. Richet, C. 1930. Une méthode générale pour mesurer l'action toxique des sesl métalliques sur la vie des organismes inférieurs. *Archives Internationale de Pharmacodynamique et de Therapie*, 38:633–35.

709. Richet, C. 1930. L'oeuvre de Marey. *Bulletin Academie de Médecine* Paris: 103:705–714 (24 June); also *Paris Médecine.* (annexe) 2i–v (16 August) also; Jules Marey, *Riforma med.* 46:1176–80 (21 July).

710. Richet, C. 1930. Un paradoxe sur la nutrition. Jeûnes prolongés dans l'hystérie. *Médecine*, 11:657–62 (September).

711. Richet, C. 1930. L'age d'or et l'age de l'or. Paris: *Editions Montaigne*.

712. Richet, C. 1930. L'anaphylaxie. Paris: F. Alcan, 328.

713. Richet, C. 1930. Pour la paix. Paris: G. Flicker, 292.

714. Richet, C. 1930. Story of civilization through the ages; foreword by Sir Oliver Lodge; translated by F. Rothwell. London: G. Allen, 115.

715. Richet, C. 1930. Foreword to Laroche, G., Richet, C. fils: and f. Saint-Girons (translated by Mildred P. and Albert H. Rowe), Berkeley: University of California Press.

716. Richet, C. 1931. Acquired psychic reflexes. *French Médicale Revue*, 1:61–63.

717. Richet, C. 1931. L'avenir et la prémonition. Paris: Montaigne, 2–48.

718. Richet, C. 1931. Les rayons cosmiques. *Revue Métapsychique*, 3:208–9.

719. Richet, C. 1931. Eugène Gley (1857–1930). *Journal de Physiologie et de Pathologie Génerale*, 29:106 (March).

720. Richet, C. 1931., Sr., and Richet, C., Jr. 1931. *Physiologie de l'homme*, Paris: Rieder, 96.

721. Richet, C. 1932. Autobiography (Le Professeur Charles Richet; autobiographie). *Biographie Médecine*, Paris: 6:145 (July), 161 (August).

722. Richet, C. 1932. Pierre Teisser. *Journal de Physiologie et de Pathologie Génerale*, Paris: 30: i–ii (June).

723. Mobrun, A., Richet, C., Facquet, J. 1932. Le névrite optique retro-bulbaire par sulfure de carbone. *Archives d'Ophthalmique*, 49:697–704 (November).

724. Richet, C. 1932. Les origines de la sérothérapie, Son passé - son present - son avenir. *Bulletin Académie de Médecine*, Paris: 108:1164–69 (25 October).

725. Richet, C. 1932. La mémoire organique (addition latente), anaphylaxie, etc). *Comptes rendus de l'Académie des Sciences*, Paris: 195:7–9 (4 July).

726. Richet, C. 1933. Que pensait-on XVII siécle de la baguette divionatoire. *Revue Métapsychique*, 3:159–63.

727. Richet, C. 1933. Pour le progrès de la métapsychique. *Revue Métapsychique*, 6:345–46.

728. Richet, C. 1933. Discours de M. Charles Richet. *Comptes rendus de l'Académie des Sciences*, Paris: 196:1–16.

729. Richet, C. 1933. La Grand Espérance. Paris: F. Aubier, 295.

730. Richet, C. 1934. Lucidité et probabilité: Une expérience de Forthuny, *Revue Métapsychique*, 4:256–60.

731. Richet, C. 1934. Un fait de prémonition au XVII siécle. *Revue Métapsychique*, 4:261.

732. Richet, C. 1934. Une prémonition remarquable. *Revue Métapsychique*, 4:321.

733. Richet, C. 1934. Notice nécrologique sur Jean Cantacuzène. *Comptes rendus de l'Académie des Sciences*, Paris: 198:217–18 (January).

734. Richet, C. 1934. Remarques sur la note de P. Rosenthal relative a l'embryothérapie. *Comptes rendus de l'Académie des Sciences*, Paris: 198:996 (March).

735. Lacroix, F.A.A. and C. Richet. 1934. Edouard Quénu, 1852–1933, Paris: Masson, 85.

736. Richet, C. 1934. *Souvenirs d'un Physiologiste*, Paris: J. Péyronnet & Cie.

737. Richet, C. 1935. La natalité en France et en Europe. *Bulletin Académie de Médecine*, Paris: 113: 219–226 (February), also *Strasbourg Medicine* (suppl) 95:265–268 (25 December).

738. Richet, C. 1935. Au secours. Paris: J. Peyronnet, 230.

739. Richet, C. 1936. Le traitement de l'anaphylaxie alimentaire. *Bruxelles Médecine*, 16:709–713 (8 March).

740. Portier, P. and C. Richet. 1936. Recherches sur la toxine de coelentères et les phenomenes d'anaphylaxie (Monaco): *Imprimerie de Monaco*, 24.
741. Richet, C. 1936. L'intelligence et l'homme; études de psychologie et de physiologie (2nd ed) Paris: F. Alcan, 376.
742. Richet, c. 1939. Autobiographie. *Biographies Médecine*, 5:278, edited by P. Busquet and Maurice Genty, Paris: Baillière.
743. Richet, C. 1952. Conférence Nobel sur l'anaphylaxie. *Internationale Archives Allergy*, 3:4–21.

Index of Proper Names

Subject Index